# Camberwell Assessment of Need for Mothers (CAN–M)

# Camberwell Assessment of Need for Mothers (CAN–M)

**A needs-based assessment for pregnant women and mothers with severe mental illness**

*Louise Howard*
*Katherine Hunt*
*Mike Slade*
*Veronica O'Keane*
*Trudi Seneviratne*
*Morven Leese*
*Graham Thornicroft*
*Malcolm Wiseman*

RCPsych Publications is an imprint of the Royal College of Psychiatrists,
17 Belgrave Square, London SW1X 8PG
http://www.rcpsych.ac.uk

British Library Cataloguing-in-Publication Data.
A catalogue record for this book is available from the British Library.

ISBN 978 1 904671 54 1

Distributed in North America by Balogh International Inc.

The views presented in this book do not necessarily reflect those of the Royal College of
Psychiatrists, and the publishers are not responsible for any error of omission or fact.

The Royal College of Psychiatrists is a charity registered in England and Wales (228636) and in
Scotland (SC038369).

Printed in the UK by Cromwell Press Ltd, Trowbridge, Wiltshire.

# Contents

# Acknowledgements

We would like to thank members of the advisory group (Jane Sayer, Jenny Shaieb, Alan Rushton, Carol Valinejad and Malcolm Wiseman) for their advice, the independent raters (Sophie Bellringer, John Boorman, Helen Gilburt, Deborah Featherstone and Manuela Jarrett) for their time, and all the service users and staff who participated in this project. This project was funded by the Guys and St Thomas' Charitable Foundation, South London and Maudsley Trustees and the Institute of Social Psychiatry.

# Contributors

Louise Howard    Clinical Senior Lecturer in Women's Mental Health, Section of Community Mental Health, Health Service and Population Research Department, Institute of Psychiatry, King's College London

Katherine Hunt    Research Worker, Section of Community Mental Health, Health Service and Population Research Department, Institute of Psychiatry, King's College London

Morven Leese    Reader and Statistician, Section of Community Mental Health, Health Service and Population Research Department, Institute of Psychiatry, King's College London

Veronica O'Keane    Clinical Senior Lecturer and Head of Section of Perinatal Psychiatry, Department of Psychiatry, Institute of Psychiatry, King's College London & Consultant Psychiatrist, South London and Maudsley NHS Foundation Trust

Trudi Seneviratne    Consultant Perinatal Psychiatrist, South London and Maudsley NHS Foundation Trust

Mike Slade    Reader in Health Services Research, Section of Community Mental Health, Health Service and Population Research Department, Institute of Psychiatry, King's College London & Clinical Psychologist, South London and Maudsley NHS Foundation Trust

Graham Thornicroft    Professor of Community Psychiatry, Section of Community Mental Health, Health Service and Population Research Department, Institute of Psychiatry, King's College London & Consultant Psychiatrist, South London and Maudsley NHS Foundation Trust

Malcolm Wiseman    Consultant Child and Adolescent Psychiatrist, South London and Maudsley NHS Foundation Trust.

# Abbreviations

| | |
|---|---|
| CAN | Camberwell Assessment of Need: a family of assessment schedules, including CAN–M (S), CAN–M (R) and CAN–M (C) |
| CAN–M | Camberwell Assessment of Need for Mothers |
| CAN–M (C) | Camberwell Assessment of Need for Mothers – Clinical version |
| CAN–M (R) | Camberwell Assessment of Need for Mothers – Research version |
| CAN–M (S) | Camberwell Assessment of Need for Mothers – Short Appraisal Schedule version |
| SMI | Severe mental illness |

# Introduction

The Camberwell Assessment of Need for Mothers (CAN–M) is a needs-based assessment specifically designed for use with pregnant women and mothers with severe mental illness (SMI). The CAN–M was developed at the Institute of Psychiatry and Kings College London, and is a modified version of the Camberwell Assessment of Need (CAN) (Slade *et al*, 1999a), the most widely used needs assessment instrument in the UK and Europe. The CAN–M is the fourth variant of the CAN. Other variants have been designed to assess the needs of populations with developmental and learning disabilities (CANDID; Xenitidis *et al*, 2003), individuals with mental illness in contact with forensic services (CANFOR; Thomas *et al*, 2003), and the elderly (CANE; Orrell & Hancock, 2004).

The CAN–M comes in three versions: a long version for research, CAN–M (R); a long version for clinical purposes, CAN–M (C); and a short version to fulfil both research and clinical purposes, CAN–M (S). The fundamental properties of the CAN–M (S), CAN–M (C) and CAN–M (R) remain the same, that is, all instruments have been designed to identify the presence of health and social care needs in pregnant women and mothers with SMI. The CAN–M (S) is a brief tool that aims to establish for each need domain: (a) whether a need is present; and (b) where a need exists, whether it is currently met or unmet. If an unmet need is identified, then further investigations may be required by an appropriate individual or team using more specialised assessment techniques. If, for example, an unmet need is identified in the *Emotional demands of childcare* domain, a full assessment by a developmental psychologist may be required. The CAN–M (C) also addresses how much help is received from informal and formal supports, and includes the service user's view of services required and action(s) needed to address the service user's needs. In contrast, the CAN–M (R) further addresses the issues of help received for each need from formal and informal supports, how much help is needed by local services to meet needs, and whether the user is receiving the right type and level of help to meet her needs.

The CAN–M incorporates 26 domains of health and social care needs relevant to pregnant women and mothers with SMI. It records the views of both the service user and their keyworker. An evaluation of the instrument has established excellent interrater reliability, test–retest reliability, content validity and concurrent validity. The CAN–M can therefore be used to identify (a) individual needs in clinical settings, such as the development of Care Programme Approach care plans and local authority parenting assessments, in addition to providing (b) a research assessment of the local service provision for pregnant women with SMI and mothers at the population-based level of need.

This manual provides an introduction to the topic of needs assessment for pregnant women and mothers with SMI (Chapter 1), a review of the needs of women with SMI during pregnancy and the postnatal period (Chapter 2) and with older children (Chapter 3), a review of the impact of maternal mental illness on the developing child (Chapter 4), a description of the development of the CAN–M (Chapter 5), a guide on how to use the CAN–M (Chapters 6 and 7), and a training package for the CAN–M (Chapter 8).

# 1 Needs assessment

## Mike Slade

## Introduction

There is growing international consensus that a needs-led approach should underpin care provided to people with SMI. For instance, the Swedish Psychiatric Care Reform, introduced in 1995, emphasises the patient's and carer's experiences of their needs (Arvidsson, 2001). In Australia, the importance of individual needs assessments for informing service development and evaluation is recognised (Mental Health Branch, 1997). In the UK, the National Service Framework for Mental Health sets standards for assessing mental health needs in primary care, and for the provision of specialist mental health services for people with multiple and complex needs (Department of Health, 1999*b*).

The term 'need' is used in two broad ways: individual and population (Slade & Glover, 2001). Individual level need refers to the problems and difficulties of an individual person. In a healthcare context, these people are actual or potential users of mental health services. Population level need refer to the needs of defined segments of the population, expressed either in terms of levels of morbidity or in terms of need for particular forms of healthcare provision. This book focuses on needs at the individual level.

Attempting to assess individual needs raises several important questions. What are needs? How are they assessed? How useful is needs assessment information, once collected? Why is a specific approach for assessing the needs of pregnant women and mothers necessary? The remainder of this chapter will address these questions.

## What are needs?

At the individual level, the concept of need has been grounded in various theories. The American psychologist Maslow proposed a hierarchy of need when attempting to formulate a theory of human motivation (Maslow, 1954). His belief was that fundamental physiological needs, such as the need for food, underpin the higher needs of safety, love, self-esteem and self-actualisation. He proposed that people are motivated by the requirement to meet these needs, and that higher needs can only be met once the lower and more fundamental needs are met. This approach can be illustrated by the example of a pregnant woman who is mentally ill and homeless and who is not concerned about attending her antenatal appointments while she is cold and hungry. Maslow therefore highlights that not all needs are equal. However, not intervening to meet a need (e.g. because addressing other needs is prioritised) should be a conscious choice rather than based on ignorance. In this example it remains important to identify the need for friends, even if no help is to be provided initially. This indicates that assessment of need should be separate from decisions about interventions to provide, a fundamental principle of needs assessment which is enshrined in the National Health Service and Community Care Act (Department of Health, 1990).

Different types of need have been identified by Bradshaw (1972): felt (experienced), expressed (experienced and communicated), normative (judgement of professionals) and comparative (based on comparison with the position of other individuals or reference groups). This taxonomy indicates that different perceptions of need can exist. Bradshaw's taxonomy provides an important set of distinctions in a mental healthcare context.

Individual patients may have impoverished expectations (e.g. due to institutionalisation), and may consequently not experience felt needs in situations where other members of the population would.

Patients may not choose to express a felt need to professionals. For example, risk to children may not be disclosed because of fears that this will lead to children being taken away. Ongoing psychotic symptoms may not be acknowledged for fear that reporting voices leads to compulsory hospitalisation.

The concept of normative needs prioritises clinical judgement over other perspectives, such as that of the patient or their informal carer. The Medical Research Council (MRC) Needs for Care Assessment (NCA) Schedule (Bebbington, 1992), for example, is based on the definition of need as 'a normative concept which is to be defined by experts' (p. 107). This approach is not consistent with the aim of the 'informed patient', and may not promote active partnership between the patient and staff.

Finally, comparative need highlights the involvement of a reference group in identifying a need. The choice of reference group is a value-based choice. For example, does a patient with SMI need a mobile phone, access to the internet, or enough money to go out for a meal? The expectations (and, therefore, the identified comparative needs) are driven by cultural, political and economic values.

Overall, the Bradshaw taxonomy highlights that need is a subjective concept, and that the judgement of whether a need is present or not will, in part, depend on whose viewpoint is being taken. There can be differences in perception between, for instance, the mental health patients and their involved professionals. If differences are identified, then it becomes possible for negotiation between staff and patient to take place so as to agree to a care plan.

Stevens & Gabbay (1991) have distinguished need (the ability to benefit in some way from healthcare), demand (wish expressed by the service user) and supply of services. These concepts can be illustrated by different components of mental health services. For instance, mental health services for people who are mentally ill and homeless are rarely demanded by people who are homeless, but most professionals would agree that a need exists. In contrast, the demand for counselling services frequently outstrips supply.

## Approaches to needs assessment

There is no perfect individual needs assessment tool. The requirements of different contexts vary, and there is inevitable conflict between factors such as brevity and comprehensiveness. Numerous approaches to assessment of need have been developed by individual teams around the country to aid care planning and reviews. There is little consistency in the information that is collected, with a tendency to concentrate on qualitative, rather than quantitative, data. Psychometric properties are frequently ignored. Although the development of such instruments help to focus a team's approach, they do not provide valid or accurate information to service planners.

One well-established needs assessment approach is the Camberwell Assessment of Need (CAN) (Phelan *et al*, 1995), which is the focus of this book. Other carefully designed needs assessment instruments include:

### 1. MRC Needs for Care Assessment (NCA)

The NCA was designed to identify areas of remediable need (Brewin *et al*, 1987). Need is defined as being present when (a) a patient's functioning (social disablement) falls below or threatens to fall below some minimum specified level, and (b) this is due to a remediable, or potentially remediable, cause. A need is defined as being met when it has attracted an item of care that is at least partly effective, and when no other item of care of greater potential effectiveness exists. A need is said to be unmet when it has only attracted a partly effective or no item of care, and when other items of care of greater potential effectiveness exist. The NCA has proved itself to be a robust research instrument, and there is a substantial body of research describing its use (Brewin *et al*, 1988; Lesage *et al*, 1991; van Haaster *et al*, 1994; O'Leary & Webb, 1996). However, it is probably too complex and time consuming for routine clinical use, and difficulties have arisen when it has been used among long-term in-patients (Pryce & Griffiths, 1993) and those who are mentally ill and homeless (Hogg & Marshall, 1992).

## 2. Cardinal Needs Schedule (CNS)

The CNS is a modification of the NCA (Marshall *et al*, 1995). It identifies cardinal problems which satisfy three criteria:

  (i)      the 'cooperation criterion' (the patient is willing to accept help for the problem);
  (ii)     the 'co-stress criterion' (the problem causes considerable anxiety, frustration or inconvenience to people caring for the patient);
  (iii)    the 'severity criterion' (the problem endangers the health or safety of the patient, or the safety of other people).

A computerised version known as AUTONEED is also available. Its use has been evaluated in routine clinical settings (Lockwood & Marshall, 1999; Marshall *et al*, 2004).

## 3. Bangor Assessment of Need Profile (BAN–P)

The BAN–P comprises a self-report schedule designed to give a brief and simple indication of the expressed need of people with a long-term mental illness, and a schedule to assess need as perceived by a key informant (Carter et al, 1996). Need is present when an item falls below that which the respondent (user or key informant) perceives to be normal or ordinary functioning, and is absent when the respondent perceives normal and independent functioning. Reliability is explored, and the instrument is primarily intended for research use.

## 4. Avon mental health measure

The Avon measure is an approach to mental health needs assessment that has been developed by Mind, a national mental health charity (Markovitz, 1996). It assesses need in 25 domains identified by mental health service users as important, and is completed by the service user, possibly with help from an advocate or care worker as necessary (Lelliott, 2000). It appears to offer some advantages over staff-rated or unstandardised assessments (Hunter *et al*, 2004), but its psychometric properties have not yet been published.

# Development of the adult Camberwell Assessment of Need (CAN)

The adult CAN was originally developed for use with adults of working age (16–65 years) with SMI. Four broad principles governed the development of the adult CAN. First, everyone has needs, and although people with SMI have some specific needs, the majority of their needs are similar to those of people who do not have a mental illness, such as having somewhere to live, something to do and enough money. Second, the majority of people with an SMI have multiple needs, and it is vital that all of them are identified by those caring for them. Therefore a priority in the adult CAN is to identify, rather than describe in detail, serious needs. Specialist assessments can be conducted in specific areas if required, once the need is identified. Third, needs assessment should be both an integral part of routine clinical practice and a component of service evaluation, so the adult CAN should be useable by a wide range of staff. Lastly, the adult CAN is based on the principle that need is a subjective concept, and that there will frequently be differing but equally valid perceptions about the presence or absence of a specific need. The adult CAN therefore records the views of staff, service users and carers separately.

The original criteria that were established for the adult CAN are that it:

(a)   has adequate psychometric properties
(b)   can be completed within 30 minutes
(c)   can be used by a wide range of professionals
(d)   is suitable for both routine clinical practice and research
(e)   can be learnt and used, without formal training
(f)   incorporates the views of both service users and staff about needs
(g)   measures both met and unmet need
(h)   measures the level of help received from friends or relatives as well as from statutory services.

The psychometric properties of the adult CAN were published in 1995 (Phelan *et al*, 1995), and have been further investigated and shown to be adequate in subsequent studies (e.g. Andresen *et al*, 2000; McCrone *et al*, 2000; Arvidsson, 2003).

Three versions of the adult CAN exist. The CAN – Research (CAN–R) is intended primarily for research use. The CAN – Clinical (CAN–C) is primarily for clinical use. The CAN Short Appraisal Schedule (CANSAS) is suitable for both research and routine clinical use. Each version of the adult CAN assesses 22 domains of health and social needs, shown in Box 1.

The adult CAN has been translated into 23 other languages, and is now the most widely reported approach to needs assessment internationally (Evans *et al*, 2000). It has been published as a book (similar in format to this volume), which contains all three versions in a form suitable photocopying, along with training and scoring materials (Slade *et al*, 1999a). Purchasing the adult CAN book allows unlimited use

---

**Box 1** Domains assessed by the adult CAN

| | |
|---|---|
| 1. Accommodation | 12. Alcohol |
| 2. Food | 13. Drugs |
| 3. Looking after the home | 14. Company |
| 4. Self-care | 15. Intimate relationships |
| 5. Daytime activities | 16. Sexual expression |
| 6. Physical health | 17. Childcare |
| 7. Psychotic symptoms | 18. Basic education |
| 8. Information on condition and treatment | 19. Telephone |
| 9. Psychological distress | 20. Transport |
| 10. Safety to self | 21. Money |
| 11. Safety to others | 22. Benefits |

for research, clinical or teaching purposes. Further information about the adult CAN is available from www.iop.kcl.ac.uk/prism/can.

## Adult CAN research

What has research using the adult CAN shown? Some features of the adult CAN were driven by prescient policy. The emphasis on the patient perspective allows explicit comparison of the staff and patient perspective on the same scale, a feature not present in other assessments. Similarly, the emphasis on needs, rather than needs for care, broke free from the restricted approach of considering only those areas of life in which mental health services have expertise, such as symptomatology and social functioning. The adult CAN domain of sexual expression illustrates this point, since it is not always routinely assessed despite the evidence for higher rates of sexual dysfunction in schizophrenia (MacDonald *et al*, 2003). Overall, some consistent findings have emerged from CAN research (in decreasing order of certainty):

1.  Patient and staff assessments of need differ (e.g. Wiersma *et al*, 1998; Lasalvia *et al*, 2000; Hansson *et al*, 2001), and patient assessments are more reliable than staff assessments (Slade *et al*, 1999*b*).
2.  Level of need is cross-sectionally associated with quality of life (UK700 Group, 1999; Hansson *et al*, 2003).
3.  The cross-sectional association with quality of life is stronger for patient-rated unmet need than staff-rated unmet need (Slade *et al*, 1999*b*; Hansson *et al*, 2003).
4.  Changes in patient-rated unmet need temporally precede changes in quality of life (Slade *et al*, 2004, 2005), indicating that needs cause quality of life.
5.  A similar causal relationship exists between patient-rated unmet need and therapeutic alliance (Junghan *et al*, 2007).

Specifically in relation to mothers, seminal work by our group has characterised the needs of mothers with psychotic disorders (Howard *et al*, 2001). For this client group, there was no significant difference in the total number of met needs rated by the patient and by staff, although patients rated higher levels of unmet need than staff. There was strong evidence that women with children were more likely than women without children to rate themselves as having a problem with intimate relationships. Patients with a history of having a looked-after child were more likely to have problems with childcare and basic education. However, this research also highlighted the need for a specific instrument to measure the needs of mothers with psychotic disorders as the available instruments did not measure some of their specific needs.

The adult CAN is used routinely in many services internationally (e.g. in Australia, England, Italy, Scotland, Spain, Sweden). Most routine uses of the adult CAN are driven by local requirements to introduce needs assessment, and are not formally evaluated. The impact is therefore difficult to judge. Formal evaluations of the impact of routine use of the CAN (Slade, 2002; Slade *et al*, 2006) and its variants (Ashaye *et al*, 2003; van Os *et al*, 2004) are only just becoming available, and research investigating the routine use of CAN in typical clinical services will be a high priority in the future.

## The need for CAN variants

In addition to the different versions of the adult CAN (CAN–R, CAN–C, CANSAS), it has been necessary to develop variants for use with other client groups. Three variants have been published.

The CAN for Developmental and Intellectual Disabilities (CANDID) is intended for use with adults with learning disabilities and mental health problems (Xenitidis *et al*, 2000), and has been published in book form (Xenitidis *et al*, 2003). The CAN – Forensic (CANFOR) is for use with people with mental health problems who are in contact with the criminal justice system ('mentally disordered offenders') (Thomas *et al*, 2008), and is available in book form (Thomas *et al*, 2003). The CAN – Elderly (CANE) is for use with older adults with mental health problems (Reynolds *et al*, 2000), and has also been published in book form (Orrell & Hancock, 2004). Each variant has been developed to be consistent with the adult CAN, but with new or amended domains which are particularly relevant to the specific client group.

There is a need for a CAN variant that particularly assesses the needs of women who have mental health problems and are pregnant and/or mothers. To justify this assertion, some of the specific needs of this client group are outlined in the next three chapters. The development of the CAN variant for pregnant women and mothers with mental health problems is then described. The overall aim is to add to the existing family of CAN assessments, to ensure that the needs of mothers and pregnant women are not neglected.

# 2 The needs of women with mental health problems during pregnancy and the postnatal period

## *Louise Howard and Veronica O'Keane*

Pregnancy is a time of physiological and emotional change for all women and these changes have particularly important consequences for women with enduring mental health problems. Psychiatric disorders are a leading cause of death during the perinatal period (pregnancy and up to 1 year post-partum) (Oates, 2000; Confidential Enquiry into Maternal and Child Health (CEMACH), 2004; Lewis, 2007). Women with chronic mental disorders who become pregnant are at high risk of obstetric complications with poorer outcomes for their babies, including low birth weight, intrauterine growth retardation, preterm birth, stillbirth and perinatal death (Bennedsen *et al*, 1999, 2001; Howard *et al*, 2003; Jablensky *et al*, 2005; Webb *et al*, 2005). This may be due to genetic susceptibility, poorer antenatal care or lifestyle factors (e.g. smoking, substance misuse, poor nutrition and socio-economic factors) (Howard, 2005). Psychotropic drugs may also have an effect on obstetric complications (in addition to the more common concern of teratogenicity), but no clinical controlled trials exist, with the few studies in the literature tending to be small with little information on confounders and drug dosage (Webb *et al*, 2004). There is some evidence that women with more common and less severe mental health problems, such as depression, tend to have shorter pregnancies and obstetric complications (Alder *et al*, 2007), though a recent meta-analysis examining anxiety symptoms during pregnancy and perinatal outcomes found no evidence of an association (Littleton *et al*, 2007); more research is needed to clarify the impact of depression and anxiety disorders on pregnancy. There is accumulating evidence though that severe psychological stress has an adverse effect on foetal development that is probably mediated through excessive stress hormone production in the mother. These stress hormones cross the placenta, inhibiting foetal growth and causing early delivery of the baby from an environment perceived as stressful. Severe psychological stress is now generally acknowledged as a common cause of preterm birth and/or low birth weight (O'Keane *et al*, 2006)

It is therefore clear that women with chronic mental health problems have specific obstetric treatment needs in addition to psychiatric treatment needs during the perinatal period. It is also well-recognised that mothers with SMI can have difficulties parenting, sometimes leading to loss of custody with mental health and emotional consequences of this for mothers and their families (Howard *et al*, 2003*b*; Howard *et al*, 2004). Many different health professionals come into contact with women with mental health problems during pregnancy and in the immediate post-partum period, providing many opportunities for intervention to prevent potentially serious sequelae. This chapter reviews the specific needs of women with mental health problems during pregnancy and in the early postnatal period.

## Obstetric care in women with severe mental illness

Women with psychiatric disorders are less likely to receive adequate antenatal care than other women (Kelly *et al*, 1999). There is evidence from the USA that women with psychotic disorders book themselves in for antenatal care later than other women (Goodman & Emory, 1992), though this has not been a consistent finding internationally (Howard *et al*, 2003a), and women with SMI may attend antenatal care less regularly than other women (Wrede *et al*, 1980; Miller & Finnerty, 1996). Yet these pregnancies are high-risk pregnancies which need optimal antenatal care. Patients with schizophrenia are at increased risk of impaired glucose tolerance and incident diabetes, particularly if they are taking atypical antipsychotic drugs (Kornegay *et al*, 2002; Lindemayer *et al*, 2003), and consequently at high risk of developing gestational diabetes. Women with chronic mental health problems are also more likely to be malnourished owing to self-neglect and/or substance misuse, and there is growing evidence that women with psychiatric disorders are more likely to smoke and misuse alcohol during pregnancy (Bennedsen *et al*, 1999; Howard *et al*, 2003a; Shah & Howard, 2006). However, general practitioners are less likely to record alcohol and smoking consumption during pregnancy in women with psychotic disorders (Howard *et al*, 2003a), suggesting that healthcare professionals may focus on the patient's psychiatric disorder to the neglect of important aspects of obstetric care. Antenatal care for women with psychotic disorders should therefore include support for women to reduce risk factors for poor perinatal outcome, including tobacco use, substance misuse, malnutrition and obesity.

Treatment needs are very complex during pregnancy and consideration about treatment when breastfeeding also needs to be taken into account at this time. Women with chronic psychiatric disorders and healthcare professionals may be concerned about possible adverse effects of prescribed drugs on the foetus during pregnancy and in the past many women have had their medication stopped during pregnancy for this reason. The pragmatic use of psychological interventions is altered by pregnancy and breastfeeding, in terms of availability, ease of access and the patient's capacity (increased physical demands and child care demands). However, not providing pharmacological or psychological treatment may produce more risks than benefits. In addition to behavioural disturbance which may put the mother and foetus at risk, it is possible that physiological changes associated with psychosis and affective disorders (e.g. increase in arousal, higher anxiety levels) could impact on the development of the foetus. Untreated psychiatric disorders may effect foeto–placental integrity and foetal central nervous system development (Cohen & Rosenbaum, 1998). It may therefore be necessary to change the type of treatment or change the treatment regimen to stabilise the mental state while avoiding foetal damage (see below). A collaborative review of illness history should include a risk–benefit assessment of treatment options.

A number of principles should guide the practice of clinicians treating women with psychotropic medication who are considering pregnancy, are pregnant or are in the postnatal period (National Institute for Health and Clinical Excellence (NICE), 2007). First, the individual women's views are key in decisions about treatment. A history of previous treatment response should be used to help guide treatment decisions and the lowest effective dose should be used if medication is thought to be necessary. Monotherapy should be used rather than combination treatments, and the balance of risks and benefits of pharmacological treatment may favour the prompt provision of psychological therapy instead. Changes in medication may be considered to reduce the risk of harm, but the risks should be balanced against the disadvantages of switching medication. Risks and benefits should be discussed with patients, partners and families in order to collaboratively agree on a care plan.

About 50% of women with a history of serious affective disorder, either recurrent depression or bipolar disorder, relapse during pregnancy (Viguera *et al*, 2000; Cohen *et al*, 2006). Findings from a study that followed about 200 women with recurrent depression through pregnancy have demonstrated that rates of relapse are 68% in those who discontinue medication following conception, compared with 26% in those who do not discontinue their mediation (Cohen *et al*, 2006). There is a general consensus that women at high risk of relapse of affective episodes (i.e. with a history of unipolar or bipolar disorder) should be particularly carefully counselled about the risks of discontinuing medication during pregnancy, although the balance of risks and benefits will vary and treatment plans should be individualised (Bonari *et al*, 2004; NICE, 2007).

Current evidence suggests that of the mood stabilisers available, lithium, while associated with a significantly increased risk of teratogenicity and, in particular, cardiac malformations, is a less harmful choice is the safest choice during pregnancy. Antipsychotic medication has been recommended by NICE (2007) as a safer alternative. The risks and benefits of switching medication, the nature of the illness and the previous response to treatment should all be considered when considering the use of mood stabilisers in pregnancy. At present, NICE recommends that pregnant women should not generally be prescribed valproate, carbamazepine, lamotrigine or paroxetine, and patients who are breastfeeding should not be routinely prescribed lithium, lamotrigine, citalopram or fluoxetine (NICE, 2007). The evidence base for prescribing in pregnancy is limited and women need to be given up-to-date information on the risks and benefits of psychotropic medication during pregnancy.

With regard to women with schizophrenia, the evidence indicates that treatment with antipsychotic medication confers either no risk or a small non-specific risk for organ malformations (Diav-Citrian *et al*, 2005). The risks of relapse may be high for women with a diagnosis of schizophrenia who discontinue medication during pregnancy (Trixler *et al*, 2005), as are the rates of voluntary termination of pregnancies. The aim for the clinician should be to provide the best information available regarding the scope of possible risks associated with the treatment of schizophrenia during pregnancy. On the basis of the available data, generalisation is impossible and recommendations should be made on an individual basis. However, clozapine should not be routinely prescribed for women who are pregnant because of the theoretical risk of agranulocytosis in the foetus, or for women who are breastfeeding, as it reaches high levels in breast milk. Depot antipsychotics also should not be routinely prescribed to pregnant women because there is little information on their safety and the infants may show extrapyramidal symptoms several months after administration of the depot (NICE, 2007); however, pregnant women who have severe illnesses that have been treated effectively by a depot or clozapine with a high risk of relapse if the medication is changed will usually need to remain on their current medication. Some women with SMI may not be well enough to effectively weigh the risks of treatment with antipsychotic medication against the risks of illness exacerbation if untreated.

Women with severe mental health problems are at increased risk of domestic violence (Post *et al*, 1980; Cascardi *et al*, 1996; Dienemann *et al*, 2000) that may start or increase in severity during pregnancy (Gazmararian *et al* 1996; Bowen *et al*, 2005). Domestic violence during pregnancy is associated with considerable physical and psychological morbidiy, and a risk of death of the mother, foetus, or both, from trauma (Amaro *et al*, 1990; Pearlman *et al*, 1990; Martin *et al*, 1998; El Kady *et al*, 2005). The Department of Health recommends routine enquiry about domestic violence, but at present most women are not routinely asked about domestic violence during pregnancy (Clark *et al*, 2000; Foy *et al*, 2000, Renker & Tonkin, 2006). Many women need to be asked about violence several times before they feel sufficiently comfortable to discuss it and are more likely to disclose domestic violence to health professionals who are supportive, non-judgemental and who ask questions in a sensitive manner (Rodriguez *et al*, 1996; Bacchus *et al*, 2003). However, there is good evidence to suggest that very few women are angry, embarrassed or offended when asked about domestic violence (Renker & Tonkin, 2006).

## Labour

There is a significantly increased risk of lack of detection of labour in women with schizophrenia compared with women with bipolar disorder (Spielvogel & Wile, 1992), which may contribute to obstetric complications in women who do not get appropriate help during labour. In women taking lithium, care needs to be taken to monitor and maintain hydration during labour as the changes in the mother's blood volume can lead to lithium toxicity in the mother and/or infant.

## Perinatal deaths

There is evidence from a recent meta-analysis of a two-fold increased risk of stillbirth in women with psychotic disorders (Webb *et al*, 2005) and there is also evidence of an increased risk of neonatal deaths

(Howard *et al,* 2003*a*), particularly in women with affective disorders and substance misuse (Webb *et al*, 2006). This is likely to be due to lifestyle factors such as smoking and substance misuse, and may also reflect the poor condition of infants at birth of women with schizophrenia who tend to have a lower Apgar score (Bennedsen *et al*, 2001). Attempted suicide during pregnancy is also associated with neonatal and infant death (Gandhi *et al*, 2006).

## Infanticide

A child under 1 year of age is four times more likely to be the victim of homicide than is a person of any other age (Marks & Kumar, 1993). Severe mental illness is directly implicated in only a minority of cases (Flynn et al, 2007), but there is an important association between fatal child maltreatment and parental psychotic disorder (d'Orban, 1979; Falkov, 1996). Less is known about more widespread but non-fatal harm or neglect of infants.

## Psychiatric complications post-partum

Women with bipolar disorder have an approximately 23-fold higher risk of admission for a primary episode (Munk-Olsen *et al*, 2006) and increased risk for recurrent episodes in puerperal women, compared with non-post-partum and non-pregnant women (Terp & Mortensen, 1998). Post-partum psychosis is a clinical variant of an episode of bipolar disorder that occurs typically in the first few days following delivery of a baby and is characterised by confusion, perplexity, fleeting psychotic beliefs and false perceptions, typically auditory, visual and tactile. Mood tends to either be manic or mixed, i.e. rapidly changing from an elated to a depressed mood or elements of both mood states present concurrently (Pfulmann *et al*, 1998). Unlike other psychoses it develops very rapidly, over a few hours or a day at the most and if untreated can often result in suicide and neonaticide. It occurs in 50% of women with a history of bipolar disorder and in 70% with a further family history of post-partum psychosis (Jones & Craddock, 2001). Women presenting with this psychosis need to be assessed rapidly and treated aggressively with antipsychotic and mood-stabilising medication. There is a further increase in risk if there is a history of a post-partum mood episode after a first pregnancy (Freeman *et al*, 2002). Women with psychotic disorders may also be at increased risk of postnatal depression compared with controls (Howard *et al*, 2004). Postnatal psychiatric care should therefore focus on relapse prevention. The mother's mental state will need to be closely monitored so that a relapse of psychosis or affective disorder can be treated quickly.

Psychiatric disorders are a leading cause of maternal death in the first year post-partum (CEMACH, 2004; Lewis, 2007). Sixty-eight per cent of maternal suicides in the first year appear to be due to psychosis or severe depressive illness (Oates, 2000), although better management of acute post-partum illnesses may improve outcome (Oates, 2000). Post-partum psychosis often presents within the first few days post-partum (Heron *et al*, 2007) when a mother may still be on the obstetric ward; however, careful monitoring of the mental state is also needed when the woman goes home with her baby.

## Parenting outcomes

Many women are able to rear a family successfully despite the presence of severe and enduring psychoses: motherhood can be a very important role for them (Krumm & Becker, 2006). However, psychotic disorders may make it hard for women to parent for a number of reasons: for example, antipsychotic medications that control symptoms may reduce responsiveness to children; withdrawal, delusional thinking and inappropriate behaviour when they occur can impair daily living and consistent parenting. Women with mental illness may also be less able to attend to their infant's physical needs such as immunisation (Howard *et al*, 2003*a*). Even women with milder psychiatric disorders, such as mild to moderate depression, have difficulties forming emotional attachments with their children; these children are disadvantaged in terms of cognitive, behavioural and emotional development relative to their peers throughout their childhood.

Mothers admitted to a psychiatric perinatal unit are more likely to have significant parenting difficulties if they have a diagnosis of schizophrenia, belong to a low social class or have a partner with a psychiatric illness (Howard *et al*, 2003*b*). Social and illness factors are therefore clearly important in parenting. Neonatal complications are also associated with problems in practical baby care and perceived risk of harm to a child in women with psychosis (Howard *et al*, 2003*b*), though it should be noted that neonatal complications are associated with bonding problems in many parents (Feldman *et al*, 1999; Poehlmann & Fiese, 2001). Fear of custody loss is a central issue in the lives of these mothers (Krumm & Becker, 2006), and when custody loss occurs women understandably suffer considerable emotional distress (Dipple *et al*, 2002; Savvidou *et al*, 2003; Sands *et al*, 2004).

Health and social services are often asked to evaluate the parenting skills of women with psychotic disorders. In cases where there is strong concern about a pregnant woman's potential parenting skills, social services should be contacted for a prebirth case conference to plan parenting assessments post-partum. Parenting assessments can take place in the community, but if there is serious concern about potential risks to the baby, such assessments can be carried out on an in-patient perinatal unit (these units are available in some parts of the UK, France and other European countries, though there are few in the USA). However, at present, services do not always make assessments optimally – in a study of mothers in a psychiatric mother and baby unit in south London where there had been pre-birth concern, pre-birth planning, in the form of a case conference and arrangements for residential assessment, occurred in less than half of admissions (Seneviratne *et al*, 2001).

## Postnatal care
### *Contraception*

Women with psychotic disorders are less likely than controls to have a record of a discussion about contraception in the first year post-partum (Rudolph *et al*, 1990; Howard *et al*, 2003*a*), even though unplanned pregnancies are more common in women with SMI (Coverdale & Aruffo, 1989; Buist *et al*, 1990). Obstetric services, psychiatric services and primary care should ensure contraceptive advice is given to these vulnerable patients (if necessary, repeatedly), as a woman who is acutely psychotic may not be responsive to her own needs. Healthcare professionals caring for chronic mental health problems need to discuss contraception needs regularly throughout the childbearing years.

## Conclusions

Many women with chronic mental health problems have children and their pregnancies are high-risk, with an increased incidence of obstetric and psychiatric complications. Pregnant women with psychoses are more likely to smoke and misuse substances than other childbearing women and they therefore need to be counselled on the risks to the baby, and given help to reduce their intake of these and other substances if possible. Optimal perinatal care frequently will also include psychotropic medication for women with chronic mental health problems, close monitoring of the patient's mental state, obstetric intervention to prevent obstetric complications, and psychiatric management of any psychiatric episodes during pregnancy and in the post-partum period. Health and social care needs of these vulnerable women should therefore be assessed regularly by healthcare professionals during pregnancy and post-partum.

# 3 The needs of severely mentally ill mothers with children

*Louise Howard and Katherine Hunt*

## Introduction

Until recently, the majority of research on mothers with SMI has focused almost exclusively on the impact of the illness on the child, whilst neglecting the needs of the mother (Gopfert *et al*, 1996). As a result, researchers and clinicians often ignore the primacy of the parenting role for these women (Bassett *et al*, 1999; Krumm & Becker, 2006), the common challenges that these women face juggling the complex demands of parenting and mental illness (Mowbray *et al*, 1995; Sands, 1995), and the level of resources required to meet basic needs, maximise parenting competency, and improve quality of life (Mowbray *et al*, 2001).

Service development and delivery in the UK to meet the needs of mothers with SMI has also received little consideration. Efforts are being made, however, to rectify this long-term neglect, as demonstrated through the publication of such reports as *Women's Mental Health: Into the Mainstream* (Department of Health, 2002) and *Mainstreaming Gender and Women's Mental Health* (Department of Health, 2003), which outline long-term plans for improving gender sensitivity and gender specificity of services. In particular, the prioritisation of service delivery for women with needs in the areas of perinatal mental health, self-harming behaviours, substance misuse, and those who experience violence and abuse, are a key focus in these reports.

In this chapter, SMI will be defined as including schizophrenia, schizoaffective disorder, bipolar disorder, and chronic affective and anxiety disorders. This chapter will discuss research into the needs of mothers with SMI, though there has been surprisingly little research in this area. This is partly because there have been no gender-sensitive instruments with which to assess the needs of mothers with SMI. This chapter therefore includes few quantitative data on women's needs and so will primarily focus on qualitative studies.

## Characteristics of mothers with severe mental illness

Before de-institutionalisation, the reproductive lives of women with SMI were often neglected. Expressions of sexuality in hospitals were often denied or ignored, with any resulting children removed from the mothers' care and put up for adoption (Apfel & Handel, 1993). Today, however, with the community as the primary focus for patient care, there is a growing recognition that women with a diagnosis of SMI are likely to be sexually active (Coverdale & Aruffo, 1989), and that the role of motherhood is a viable option (Apfel & Handel, 1993).

Studies by our and other research groups across different Westernised populations have shown that the majority of women with SMI have children (McGrath *et al*, 1999; Howard *et al*, 2001). We have reported that the fertility of women with SMI, particularly schizophrenia, is significantly lower than the general population (Howard *et al*, 2002) but with the advent of atypical antipsychotic drugs, which do not cause hyperprolactinaemia, this is likely to rise. Women with SMI who have children tend to have higher levels of functioning compared with other women with SMI who do not have children; for example, they are significantly older, have an older age of illness onset, and are more likely to live in unsupported accommodation (Howard *et al*, 2001).

The actual percentage of mothers, however, who manage to retain primary custody of their children has been reported with remarkably variable rates, differing depending on the setting, research methods and sampling techniques used. For example, Dipple *et al* (2002) found that of 58 women at rehabilitation services in Leicester who had children, 68% were permanently separated from at least one child before the age of 18 years and often had little or no subsequent contact with them. Similarly, Joseph *et al* (1999) found that only 21% of severely ill mothers hospitalised in an American inner-city facility had retained full custody of their children, whereas other studies have identified even smaller primary custody rates of around 9% (White *et al*, 1995).

In a longitudinal study of mothers with SMI in Michigan, Hollingsworth (2004) reported that mothers who lose custody of their children tended to be single, had never married, had a longer duration of mental illness, experienced more hospitalisations, and often had incomes below the poverty line. The likelihood of custody loss was also found to increase with each additional child and additional psychiatric hospitalisation. However, custody loss was less likely if a woman perceived motherhood as being a personal benefit to her life, her income was above the poverty level, and if she had support with childcare.

Custody loss appears to be more likely in women with a diagnosis of schizophrenia compared with mood disorders (White *et al*, 1995; Howard *et al*, 2004) and in women from Black and minority ethnic groups (Sands, 1995; Howard *et al*, 2001), though this is not a consistent finding (White *et al*, 1995). These findings may be explained by confounding factors such as the presence of a partner.

## The experience of motherhood

A number of qualitative studies have investigated the experiences and needs of mothers with SMI. Many of these studies have identified needs that are similar to those mothers without mental illness, particularly those relating to the normal hassles of everyday parenting. That is, mothers with SMI are able to identify both rewarding and troublesome aspects of motherhood, and just like any other mothers, may sacrifice their own needs to meet the perceived needs of their children (Nicholson *et al*, 1998a). Similarly, many women, including in-patients, describe their children as being the primary source of joy in their life (Savvidou *et al*, 2003; Diaz-Caneja & Johnson, 2004). Pride derived from parenthood was also found to be a powerful motivating force in recovering from illness and an incentive to remain well in the hope that the children would be returned to their care (Nicholson *et al*, 1998a; Diaz-Caneja & Johnson, 2004).

However, a number of burdensome aspects of parenting in the context of SMI bring significant stress to the lives of women who are mentally ill. In particular, studies have found that mothers with mental illness often have problems in the areas of medication side-effects, for example sedation (Nicholson *et al*, 1998a; Savvidou *et al*, 2003); buying food and preparing appropriate meals (Howard *et al*, 2001); fears surrounding the loss of custody (Bassett *et al*, 1999; Krumm & Becker, 2006), including voluntary placements when they are hospitalised (Nicholson *et al*, 1998a); and anxieties regarding the impact of their illness on their children such as feelings of guilt about what they may have 'done wrong' (Nicholson *et al*, 1998a).

Concerns about stigma can prevent women from talking openly about the difficulties they experience (Diaz-Caneja & Johnson, 2004; Thornicroft, 2006), their willingness to seek help and engage in treatment (Ackerson, 2003), and fear that people may treat them and their children differently if they knew about the mental illness (Bassett *et al*, 1999). Parents who have gone through a divorce often report having their diagnosis used against them while fighting for custody in the courts (Ackerson, 2003).

The trauma of hospitalisation is also a major concern for mothers with SMI (Bassett *et al*, 1999; Diaz-Caneja & Johnson, 2004). Several participants in focus groups stated that in-patient units were inappropriate places for children to visit them, primarily due to the behaviour of the other patients and the lack of adequate facilities such as family visiting rooms separated from the main ward (Diaz-Caneja & Johnson, 2004). Significantly, this was thought to impact on the mothers' ability to maintain contact with their children during an admission.

# The impact of mental illness on parenting

Studies have examined the impact that a mental illness can have on a woman's ability to parent and the difficulties that women with mental illness can face in managing their children's behaviour (Sands, 1995; Nicholson *et al*, 1998*a*; Ackerson, 2003). Ackerson (2003) asked women directly about their parenting needs, and found that many of the mothers interviewed admitted to having difficulties in the area of discipline; women were more likely to see themselves as too lax or permissive than too harsh. Some expressed this as a consequence of their own perceptions of inadequacy and the guilt they felt about becoming a parent who was mentally ill. Others reported difficulties in exerting their parental authority due to the role reversal that occurred as a result of acute episodes of their illness. However, Sands (1995) found that mothers who were mentally ill tended not to acknowledge they had difficulties managing their children, while Mullick *et al* (2001) showed that better insight into mental illness was associated with more sensitive mothering behaviour and with lower risk of maltreatment.

Studies have shown that specific diagnoses may elicit certain behaviours in mothers. Weinberg & Tronick (1998) found that when observed with their children, mothers with mood and anxiety disorders were more disengaged, withdrawn or intrusive than controls. Similarly, Egami *et al* (1996) found that anxiety was associated with child neglect. Other reports have suggested that mothers with depression are likely to be more negative (Radke-Yarrow *et al*, 1993), may spend less time looking at and touching her baby, and may respond more slowly to the baby's activity (Radke-Yarrow *et al*, 1985; Stein *et al*, 1991). These behaviours can lead to anxious or avoidant attachment (see Chapter 4). Psychotic disorders may make it hard for women to parent for a number of reasons – for example, antipsychotic medications that control symptoms may reduce responsiveness to children; withdrawal, delusional thinking and inappropriate behaviour when they occur can impair daily living and consistent parenting; and there is some research documenting problems of mother–infant attachment. Mothers admitted to a psychiatric mother and baby unit are more likely to have significant parenting difficulties if they have a diagnosis of schizophrenia, belong to a low social class or have a partner with a psychiatric illness (Howard *et al*, 2003*b*). Social *and* illness factors are therefore clearly important in parenting.

Many women are able to rear families successfully despite the presence of severe and enduring psychoses – parents within any given diagnostic category can have parenting skills ranging from excellent to maltreating (Rogosch *et al*, 1992; Mowbray, *et al*, 1995), and mothers with SMI have been found to parent as well as or better than matched controls (Weinberg & Tronick, 1998). A number of factors are thought to have an impact on parenting capabilities. These include lack of effective knowledge and skills (Nicholson *et al*, 1998*b*), pre-morbid functioning and timing of illness exacerbation (Rodnick & Glodstein, 1974; Bybee *et al*, 2003), parental stress, including stresses related to the special needs of the child (Oyserman *et al*, 2002), effective social support (Nicholson *et al*, 1998*b*), and maternal poverty (Bybee *et al*, 2003; McLoyd, 1998).

Unfortunately many studies examine only the mothers' difficulties and weaknesses whilst neglecting their parenting strengths and commitment to their children. While it is true that a significant number of mothers who are mentally ill will lose custody of their children, many women are still capable of caring for their children and, as assessed by the local authorities, have 'good enough' parenting to retain primary custody. It is this particular group of women who are overlooked in the research and deserve greater attention so as to improve clinicians and researchers understanding of the factors that lead to resilience.

# Personal relationships, role of the extended family and social supports

Although women with SMI place a great deal of importance on personal relationships, they are often found to have difficulties in establishing and maintaining support networks (Ritscher *et al*, 1997). In a UK epidemiological study, we found that 29% of mothers with psychosis reported problems with starting and maintaining intimate relationships (Howard *et al*, 2001), while Mowbray *et al* (2005a, 2005b) found that the highest rated interpersonal hassle of mothers with mental illness was the children's father. Research has also shown that women with mental illness are more likely to marry a spouse with a psychiatric disorder (Rutter & Quinton, 1984), have lower marriage rates and higher divorce rates than women without mental illness (Goldman, 1982), and describe the support or assistance received from fathers as being characteristically low (Mowbray *et al*, 1995).

In a qualitative study by Nicholson *et al* (1998b), 42 mothers with mental illness were asked about their perceptions of their relationship with husband or partner. Several important themes were identified from these focus groups. Some of the women described their partner/husband as being very helpful with daily parenting tasks or emergencies, while others were seen to be passively or actively destabilising the mothers' efforts to cope with mental illness and parenting demands. Other partners/husbands were described as having unrealistic expectations of the situation, depleting the women's energy, displaying abusive behaviour towards the mother and children, and engaging in drug-taking behaviour. Case managers also spoke of the 'need' for many of the mothers to hold on to their 'well' partner/husband in order to justify retaining custody of their children to child welfare agencies, yet they could also be held responsible for their inability to protect their children if these 'well' husbands/partners were found to be violent within the home.

## Extended family

Savvidou *et al* (2003) found that the contribution of other family members to parenting (child rearing, helping with childcare, helping with daily activities or with housekeeping) could be characterised as both negative and positive. Most of the mothers said that their family members did not understand 'mental illness', and that they were often angry and judgemental towards them. Further, some family members reinforced the 'role of the invalid' and failed to consider the mother's wishes when making decisions about the children. The majority of mothers who were mentally ill (86%) living with their children, however, did identify grandparents as being significant sources of daily support for childcare. In fact, 40% of divorced mothers were primarily living with their parents so that someone would be there to help care for the children. Some grandparents, however, may be dysfunctional parents themselves, and as a result, some mothers may not fully trust the childcare provided by the grandparents (Nicholson *et al*, 1998b).

## Social networks and community support

Mothers with mental illness who care for their children have better immediate and extended social networks than do women with mental illness who do not engage in child-rearing activities (White *et al*, 1995; Howard *et al*, 2001). These mothers are still reported, however, to have poor relationships with their neighbours (Savvidou *et al*, 2003) and, in the case of mothers from Black and minority ethnic groups, may be at risk of feeling isolated and bereft of family support (Nicholson *et al*, 1998*b*). In terms of using mental health providers as sources of support, Mowbray *et al* (2000) found that while nearly all of the mothers (96%) in their study had received mental health services in the past 3 months, only 44% chose to list a mental health provider as a source of support, and even fewer (20%) listed their provider as someone who could give support and advice about being a mother.

## Economic, employment and education needs

Literature reviews have uncovered consistent findings in regards to the adverse impact that unmet accommodation, poverty and finance, education and employment needs can have on mothers and their families.

### Accommodation needs

It is well-established that mental illness is associated with housing problems and homelessness. For example, we found that 31% of mothers with psychosis rate themselves as having unmet needs in the area of accommodation (Howard *et al*, 2001). Significantly, mothers who are homeless may also lose their children to involuntary foster care placement if their inability to provide a home is perceived as neglectful (Bassuk *et al*, 1996). Once without children, they may lose welfare benefits and food tokens, further decreasing their chances of securing housing and reuniting their family. Owing to this vicious cycle, they may be unable to regain custody of their children, even in cases without prior evidence of parental abuse or neglect (Bassuk *et al*, 1996).

### Poverty, welfare benefits and budgeting

The relationship between mental health and poverty is well established, showing that individuals in lower economic groups experience higher rates of psychiatric problems than those in higher socio-economic groups (Belle, 1982; Bassuk *et al*, 1998). We found that 32% of mothers with psychosis rate themselves as having unmet needs with welfare benefits, either reporting that they do not receive the appropriate benefits or that they are uncertain as to whether they are receiving all the benefits to which they are entitled (Howard *et al*, 2001). Adjusted for family size, more than two-thirds of mothers recruited from psychiatric services in Detroit had a household income below the poverty line (Mowbray *et al*, 2000).

### Employment needs

Employment problems experienced by mothers with serious mental illness have been highlighted in a report by Mowbray *et al* (2000) which found that in a group of 379 mothers recruited from community mental health teams and in-patient units in Detroit, 78% were unemployed, compared with 18% in other women living in the same areas. In the UK, employment problems have also been highlighted in similar studies (Howard *et al*, 2001).

## Domestic violence and abuse

There has been increasing awareness of the poor health and social outcomes in women who experience domestic violence. Guidelines have been developed on how health workers can better identify, support, and refer victims of violence (Department of Health, 2006). These actions result from a growing recognition that violence is a risk factor for many physical and psychological health problems (Royal College of Psychiatrists, 2002; Watts & Zimmerman, 2002). Management of violence against women is now considered a core competency for mental health workers in the UK (Department of Health, 2006).

One of the most common forms of violence against women is that perpetrated by a husband or other intimate male partner. Intimate partner violence or domestic violence may take various forms, including physical violence (slaps, punches, assaults with a weapon) and sexual violence (forced sex or participation in degrading sexual acts). These acts are frequently accompanied by emotionally abusive behaviours such as intimidation, prohibiting a woman from seeing her family and friends, and other controlling behaviours. Women of Black and ethnic minorities who experience domestic violence are thought to be particularly vulnerable to isolation and experience many barriers to accessing help; for example, language barriers may limit their access to resources (Royal College of Psychiatrists, 2002). Recent studies internationally have highlighted the common experience of violence and abuse against women with SMI (Post *et al*, 1980; Dienemann *et al*, 2000). Violence in an adult relationship is associated with an increased risk of child abuse and children who see violent behaviour at home are more likely to suffer long-term psychological consequences, including anxiety, conduct problems and overt aggression (Moss, 2003; Wolfe *et al*, 2003). Domestic violence also impacts on maternal–foetal bonding; mothers abused during pregnancy may be less likely to bond well with their foetus and subsequently their child (Zeitlin *et al*, 1999). This can have detrimental effects on the child's social, cognitive, emotional and behavioural development (Wolfe *et al*, 2003), which will further exacerbate problems associated with deficits in parenting due to mental illness.

## Conclusion

This chapter indicates that while mothers with SMI may have a higher level of functioning than other women with SMI, their parenting role leads to particular difficulties in their everyday lives which need to be addressed by services in order to achieve optimal parenting. This is important for the mothers themselves, who see motherhood as a central role in their lives, and equally importantly it is essential for their children.

# 4 The impact of maternal mental illness on the developing child

*Malcolm Wiseman*

## Introduction

Mental health problems are common, and there is a strong association between illness in a parent and problems in their children (Rutter, 1966). The mechanisms that link parental mental illness and childhood problems are complex. Mental illness often coexists with other areas of difficulty such as poverty and low socio-economic status, stigma and discrimination, all of which can on their own or in combination impact on child development. The links between parental mental illness and these features of psychosocial disadvantage make the mechanisms by which parental mental illness affect child development difficult to disentangle; however, there is a growing body of evidence that suggests that genetic factors interact with environmental factors to determine whether a child develops a disorder, as well as the course and timing of its onset. In addition, mental ill-health can fluctuate over time in response to stresses and other factors, and despite the well-established links between parental mental illness and childhood psychiatric disorder, some children will show resilience and do not experience difficulties (Kaufman *et al*, 1979).

This chapter will review the extent of the problem and the kinds of difficulties found in children when a mother is mentally ill will be described. Child protection and safeguarding issues will also be considered and some thoughts on the mechanisms by which parental mental illness may affect children will be explored. As already stated, not all children are adversely affected by parental mental illness, and factors that promote resilience and protect children will be presented. Finally, young carers' views about their needs in relation to their ill parents will also be considered.

## The extent of the problem

The experience of living with a parent who is mentally ill is a common one. About 10% of the adult population suffer from some form of mental illness, and over a lifetime there is a one in four chance of experiencing mental illness (Thompson & Pudney, 1990; Mind, 1997). Psychiatric admission rates for women aged between 20 and 44 years (i.e. those most likely to be looking after children) represent nearly 20% of all in-patient episodes (Department of Health, 1995).

Major problems, such as bipolar disorder, schizophrenia and substance misuse, affect 1 in 40 in the population (Meltzer *et al*, 1995), mainly younger adults and the unemployed. The presence of any mental health problem (moderate or severe) was highest amongst parents (single or a couple) living with dependent children. For lone parents (mainly mothers) compared with other parents, there is a threefold increase in the likelihood of suffering from a major problem, and for moderate problems there is a twofold increase.

Brown & Harris (1978) showed that about a quarter of inner-city women with children under 5 years experienced depression following a significant life event, and that lower social class increased the vulnerability to depression, while Richman *et al* (1982) found that 30–40% of mothers looking after young children had depression. Another study (Meltzer *et al*, 1995) found that the prevalence of neurotic disorders (depression, mixed anxiety and depression, and alcoholism) was highest amongst lone parents. A US study found that 25% of all patients with serious mental illness had children, and for women under 35 years, 45% were mothers (Blanch *et al*, 1994). An epidemiologically representative cohort study of women with chronic psychotic disorders in south London reported that over 60% had had children (Howard *et al*, 2001); similar figures have been reported in Australia (McGrath *et al*, 1999). Surveys, generally, however, are likely to underestimate the number of parents with mental illness looking after children, as adult mental heath services do not routinely collect information on children or on adults as parents. The evidence therefore suggests that many children live in families where at least one parent has mental health problems, and lone parents and women are particularly vulnerable.

# Effects on children

## Emotional and behavioural

Children of parents with mental health problems are three times more likely than others to have mental health problems (Meltzer *et al*, 2000). Similarly, in a US, community-based study (Weissman *et al*, 2004), a sample of mothers presenting in primary care were screened for mental health problems. Mothers with depression reported a threefold increased risk of emotional problems in their children. Rutter & Quinton (1984) demonstrated that approximately a third of children of parents with mental illness have a persistent childhood psychiatric disorder, a third have transient disorders, while a third have no disorder, and whereas children of well parents have similar rates for transient disorders, the rate for a persistent disorder amongst the parental mental illness group was twice that for the non-parental mental illness group.

Most of the studies of the effect of parental mental illness on children have involved mothers with depression. In one such study, difficult behaviours in the children were more prevalent in parents with SMI compared with moderate depression, suggesting that severity rather than specific diagnoses might be the key factor (Lee & Gotlib, 1989).

However, parents with a psychiatric disorder experience higher rates of common risk factors for childhood psychiatric disorders, including single parenthood, separations, divorce, marital discord, parental history of being in care, parental criminality, large family size, overcrowding and poverty. This influences the presence of mental health problems in children. The risk of child problems increases with the number of areas of family difficulty, for example parental mental illness, substance misuse, domestic violence (Whitaker *et al*, 2006). Persistent marital discord, including violence in the relationship, would appear to be the most significant risk factor for the development of psychiatric disorder, especially for boys. The greater levels of psychosocial disadvantages found in families where there is parental mental illness probably accounts for much of the increased rate of childhood psychiatric disorder (Rutter & Quinton, 1984). The same study noted that the disorders in children are not linked to specific types of parental disorder, although personality disorders, probably through their association with hostile, aggressive behaviour, was the only diagnosis that increased the rate of disturbance in children.

The literature on the specificity of the links between the parental disorder and the child's disorder is mixed, but studies of less disadvantaged populations find links between specific parental diagnoses and childhood disorders. Depression and anxiety disorders were more common in children (especially girls) of parents with depression (especially mothers), and boys were more likely to develop behaviour problems when both parents had a psychiatric illness. The combination of a father who was an alcoholic and a mother with depression was particularly damaging (Foley *et al*, 2001). Children of parents with anxiety are more likely to suffer from anxiety disorders, while children of parents with depression show a broader range of disorders and frequent comorbidity (Beidel & Turner, 1997), and substance misuse in parents is associated with higher rates of conduct disorder and attention-deficit hyperactivity disorder in boys (Kuperman *et al*, 1999).

Although there are links between specific disorders in parents and specific disorders in children, there is also evidence that important mediating influences are adverse psychosocial factors present in the family, and, in particular, hostility, aggression, marital discord and disruption (Emery *et al*, 1982; Rutter, 1982). For this reason, parental personality disorders, substance misuse and the presence of domestic violence have the most detrimental influence on children.

Parental mental illness, especially maternal mental illness, may affect the attachment relationships, which in turn effects the psychological development of the child. A mother with depression may spend less time looking at and touching her baby, and may respond more slowly to the baby's activity (Radke-Yarrow *et al*; 1985; Stein *et al*, 1991). These behaviours can promote anxious or avoidant attachment in the child's second year, which can be reversed if there are improved relationships later (Ainsworth *et al*, 1978), but which can otherwise be associated with emotional and behavioural problems in later childhood, as well as relationship difficulties in adulthood. These effects of maternal depression were found to be independent of the length of the mother's illness, so interventions need to focus on the mother–child relationship and not only on treating the maternal depression (Murray *et al*, 1999). Mothers with schizophrenia were noted to be more detached and insensitive with their babies, compared with those suffering from depression, although other factors, such as the effects of drug treatment, could be contributory factors (Riordan *et al*, 1999).

In addition to the effects on children's emotional and behavioural development, parental mental illness can also adversely effect children's educational and cognitive development. Again, these studies have largely focused on the effects of maternal depression. Postnatal depression, but not antenatal or concurrent depression, impairs cognitive development at 4 years, and this is worse for boys (Coghill *et al*, 1986; Sharp *et al*, 1995). However, others have ascribed these findings not so much to the depression as to the adverse social and economic circumstances associated with depression (Kurstjens & Wolke, 2001). Cooper & Murray (1998) report an association between a disturbed mother–child relationship and an adverse impact on the child's cognitive and emotional development. Many children will have missed school because of their parent's mental illness (Aldridge & Becker, 2003), which may affect their educational achievement but which may also affect (or reflect) their emotional state, as staying away from school is often linked to worries about their parent's health and safety.

## Longer-term effects

Children of parents with mental illness have an increased risk of suffering from mental health difficulties in their own adulthood (Carlson & Weintraub, 1993) and children of parents with an affective disorder have a 40% chance of developing a major depressive disorder by the age of 20 years (Beardslee *et al*, 1998). A longitudinal study of the now adult children of mothers with depression during their offspring's childhood, which controlled for other risk factors, concluded that daughters had a two-and-a-half times greater risk of developing a depressive disorder during their lifetime (than controls) and although sons did not appear to have a greater risk of developing depression, they did show poorer educational attainment (Ensminger *et al*, 2003). Weissman *et al* (2006a), in a 20-year follow-up study of offspring of parents with and without depression, found that the risks for anxiety disorders, major depression, and substance dependence were approximately three times as high in the offspring of parents with depression as in those of parents without depression. Females were more affected, and the period of highest incidence was between the ages of 15 and 20 years. There were also higher rates of physical illness and mortality in the offspring of parents with depression.

There is a strong link between poor parenting, abuse and separations, adult personality disorder (Zeitlin, 1986), and high rates of personality problems, as well as a wide range of other difficulties, including anxiety disorders and antisocial behaviours, are found in the adult sons of parents who are alcoholics (Greenfield *et al*, 1993; Mathew *et al*, 1993).

Various mechanisms have been suggested for this link, including genetic predisposition for the major mental illnesses, as about 13% of children with one affected parent will develop schizophrenia, while 5–10% of children with one affected parent will develop bipolar disorder (with an additional risk of 10–20% of unipolar depression). Second, parental mental illness creates problems in parenting, with long-lasting effects on development (Roy, 1990) or is associated with many psychosocial adversities which also predispose to long-term difficulties for the developing child. Third, children may learn behaviour patterns and maintain these behaviours through adulthood (Focht-Birkerts & Beardslee, 2000).

## *Quality of life*

Apart from the increased rates of childhood psychiatric disorder, children also report distress about their situation and it is clear that parental mental illness has a negative effect on their quality of life. A third of parents with mental illness report a disruption to their children's normal daily life as a result of their mental illness (Stallard *et al*, 2004). For example, they may not be available to their children because of hospital appointments, they may not be available to attend school meetings because of anxieties, or they may not be able to play with their children because of depression. Children may have increased responsibilities for their parent or siblings as carers (Deardon & Becker, 2000), which may restrict their social lives and relationships, with a third of children expressing the view that their relationships with friends had changed, usually for the worse, with embarrassment, reluctance to bring friends home and feeling isolated being common themes (Stallard *et al*, 2004). In addition, children of parents with depression are more likely to express suicidal thoughts or actions (Klimes-Dougan *et al*, 1999).

## Child protection and safeguarding

Parental mental illness has a negative effect on parenting, and this can cross the threshold of significant harm which, in the UK, justifies compulsory intervention by the state as outlined in the Children's Act 1989. The harm can be to the child's emotional development or to their physical health, including physical injury or death.

A significant proportion of mothers with a major psychiatric illness lose custody of their children, particularly women with a history of psychiatric admissions (Coverdale & Aruffo, 1989; Miller & Finnerty, 1996). In various surveys (Ritsher *et al*, 1997), around half of the women with schizophrenia had had children, and half of these had had their children removed from their care. Those that retained custody often shared the care with family members, usually the maternal grandmother (Caton *et al*, 1998), involving the children in what has been termed intermittent parenting.

The ability of these mothers to look after their children will depend, in part, on the effectiveness of their treatment, their access to mental health services (including services that will address the children's needs), the support that is available (including that from family members) and reduction in stigma. Parents are often reluctant to seek help, as they fear they will lose their children (Cogan, 1998); in addition, interviews with parents with mental illness revealed that 40% had never received professional help in relation to their children, while a third had asked for help but had not received any (Wang & Goldschmidt, 1994, 1996).

In a study using focus groups of mothers with severe mental illness, the mothers were particularly concerned about disciplining their children, and found it difficult to distinguish between the effects of stress related to parenting and the effects of their illness. Some mothers avoided their medication in order to increase their sensitivity to their children. They reported that they would delay seeking help, when they became ill, for fear of losing their children (Nicholson *et al*, 1998a). It should also be noted that the emphasis on community-based adult mental health services will mean that there will be increased numbers of children living with parents who are mentally ill, for longer periods of time, with little or no support in place for them.

Parents with mental illness, or those with substance misuse, are significantly more likely to neglect or abuse their children (Browne & Herbert, 1997): in a large community sample, adults who reported a parental history of mental illness had a two- to three-fold increase in the rates of physical, sexual, or any abuse. A diagnosis in the parent of antisocial personality disorder increased the risk of physical abuse but otherwise the parental diagnosis was not correlated with the type of abuse (Walsh *et al*, 2002). However, mental illness would appear to be just one component and there is a strong association and interaction between the mental illness and socio-demographic factors, such as unemployment, poverty, and family violence, which are also associated with child abuse (Gelles, 1973). Black & Mayer (1980) studied parents who misused alcohol and opiates, comparing those who abused their children with a non-abusive sample, and found that mothers who misused substances were more likely to abuse children, that violence between the parents was one of the strongest predictors of violence between the mother and the child, and that poverty and poorer living situations were associated with child maltreatment. Children of parents abusing substances experience very negative childhoods, including high levels of violence (Black *et al*, 1986) and inconsistency (Jarmas & Kazak, 1992).

Studies from the USA (Taylor *et al*, 1991) describe high rates of schizophrenia and depression amongst parents who abuse their children, whereas UK studies describe mainly depression, personality disorders, and substance misuse (Falkov, 1997) and deliberate self-harm (Hawton *et al*, 1985), possibly reflecting different service provision and reporting arrangements.

There are some (weak) links between the parental disorder and the type of abuse. Zuravin (1988) found that current depression, as well as a past history of depression, in mothers, was significantly associated with abuse and neglect independently of socio-economic disadvantages, and Famularo *et al* (1992) found an association between alcohol misuse and physical abuse of the child, and cocaine misuse and sexual abuse of the child.

Around 200–300 children die each year as a result of child abuse and neglect in England and Wales (Wilczynski, 1994), and younger children (under the age of 2 years) are particularly at risk (Reder & Duncan, 1997). The majority die as a result of physical abuse, although neglect may also be a cause of death.

In his study of women remanded to prison for killing their children, d'Orban (1979) found that 27% of the mothers were mentally ill (psychosis, depression, or personality disorder with depression), while 10% had severe personality disorders with aggressive, impulsive behaviour and a history of many hospital admissions. Of the sample, 40% had battered their child in a sudden impulsive act – this group was not considered mentally ill at the time of the attack, but their backgrounds were characterised by violence, chaos and separations. The mentally ill group was thought to have experienced less marital stress, and two-thirds had attempted or contemplated suicide. Only in a half the women with psychosis, in this prison-based sample, was killing associated with puerperium.

More recent studies have confirmed the high prevalence (around 50%) of psychiatric illness in one or both carers where a child dies of abuse or neglect (Reder & Duncan, 1999; Wilczynski, 1995). Puerperal illness was rare in these groups, presumably because sufferers would be in close contact with services and could be treated quickly. Psychosis was found in around 10%, depression in around 20% and substance misuse in around 20–33%. Many had withdrawn from services just before causing the injury. In a small study of child deaths occurring in a mental health service, where abuse or neglect was a relevant factor in the deaths, 71% of the perpetrators were known to adult mental health services (including addictions and perinatal services), and there was a tendency for the women to harm younger children, compared with male perpetrators (Wiseman & Lewis, 2006).

## Mechanisms

Although some ideas about the mechanisms linking parental mental illness and adverse effects on children have been discussed above, these will now be considered in more detail. It should be noted, however, that many of the studies lack control groups; therefore, the links between the parent's illness and the child's adjustment are unclear and could be related to a number of factors, including the specific illness or the more general risk factors so often present, as well as the common occurrence of comorbidity.

The genetic endowment of a child will interact with environmental factors such as quality of parenting or life events to determine whether the child will develop a disorder, its severity, and the course and timing of its onset (Tienari *et al*, 1994). Genetic factors in childhood psychiatric disorders have been reviewed in Rutter *et al* (1990).

The complex nature of mental disorders means that it is difficult to identify the genes for these disorders and to define the particular environments that would allow the psychopathology to emerge. In a study of adult female twins, all the genes that influenced risk of generalised anxiety disorder and major depression were shared between the two disorders, and therefore environmental factors would largely be responsible for whether the adult woman expressed her genetic vulnerability as anxiety or depression (Kendler *et al*, 1992). Roy *et al* (1995) suggested that the type of stressful life event determines whether anxiety or depression develops, with generalised anxiety disorder being associated with life events that involve danger, while life events that involve loss are associated with the development of depression. Silberg *et al* (2001) conducted a study on adolescent girls and concluded that there is an environmentally mediated effect of life events on depression and anxiety, and that genetic factors play a significant role in individual differences in susceptibility to these environmentally mediated risks. In the absence of parental emotional disorder, the negative life events had no effect, while where there was parental disorder the life events did have a significant effect. In a three-generation study (Weissman *et al*, 2005), high rates of psychiatric disorder (especially anxiety) were found in the grandchildren of families where there were two generations suffering from major depression. Parental major depressive disorder and child diagnosis were moderated by grandparental major depression. In those families where both the grandparents and the parents suffered from depression, the grandchildren had high rates of both anxiety and any childhood psychiatric disorder. In those families where only the parent suffered from depression, there was no significant effect on the diagnosis of the grandchildren, although the presence of parental depression did have a significant impact on the grandchildren's functioning. Rates of disorder in children were highest when both parents and grandparents had depression, and for the younger children they concluded that anxiety disorders were an early sign of psychopathology.

The genetic risk can also be very specific. Family environmental factors (such as marital, legal or psychological problems) in adoptive families increased the risk of childhood aggression, adolescent aggression and conduct disorder in adopted children, but only when the biological background of the adoptees included antisocial personality disorders. There was virtually no effect of the environment on those adoptees not at genetic risk. The biological background of alcohol misuse did not interact with an adverse adoptive home environment to increase the risk of antisocial behaviour, demonstrating the specificity of the genetic predisposition for antisocial behaviour (Cadoret *et al*, 1995). Rutter & Silberg (2002) conclude that twin and adoption studies suggest that the impact of environmental risk factors on psychopathology is slight in the absence of genetic risk. A further factor to consider is the effect of the child's behaviour on the parenting environment. Children of parents with antisocial behaviour, who demonstrated antisocial behaviour, evoked harsh and inconsistent parenting in their adoptive parents (Ge *et al*, 1996; O'Connor *et al*, 1998).

The parenting behaviours of parents with mental illness can also have a direct effect on the developing brain, and the neurobiological effects of parenting are receiving attention. Prenatal factors such as maternal alcohol misuse (Fitzgerald *et al*, 2000) can harm brain development. Gunnar (1998) suggests that more optimal parenting, as evidenced by security of attachment, buffers the effects of stress on the developing brain, and electroencephalography (EEG) changes have been noted in both mothers with depression and their infants (Dawson *et al*, 1997), with relatively decreased EEG activity in the left frontal lobe (an area associated with positive emotions) as compared with activity in the right frontal lobe (associated with negative emotions such as sadness). Forbes *et al* (2006) have also found in children of parents with depression, left frontal EEG asymmetry in children with anxiety or depression and aggressive behaviour difficulties.

A further risk to the unborn child comes from sub-optimal antenatal care. Mothers who are mentally ill are more likely to have unplanned pregnancies, poorer antenatal care and far higher risks of premature or ill babies (Stewart & Gangbar, 1984), while other perinatal risk factors such as smoking, poor diet, and alcohol or substance misuse in pregnancy are also found more commonly in association with maternal mental illness (Taylor, 1991) (see also Chapter 2).

Adverse life events are associated commonly with child psychiatric disorder (Goodyer *et al*, 1985), and families with parental mental illness are exposed more commonly to a wide variety of these events. These include separations, due to, for example, hospitalisations, marital breakdown, and reception into care (Smith, 2004) unemployment and poverty (Bornstein *et al*, 2003), and bereavements (including as a result of suicide). Poor housing and disputes with neighbours are more common in the lives of mothers with depression (Cox *et al*, 1987). All these negative environmental experiences increase the risks to an already vulnerable child.

Few studies have looked at the effect of ethnicity on parenting and maternal mental illness. A recent study examined the processes by which parenting practices, maternal depression and chronic poverty affected child behavioural problems in different ethnic groups. Poverty, depression and parenting all affected child behaviour problems in the different ethnic groups. However, the processes and mechanisms through which they exert their effects differ among the groups. Poverty affected child behaviour indirectly through the other variables, while parenting practices had direct effects. The study found that the effects of maternal depression were partly mediated through parenting in the White and Latino groups, but were direct and unmediated through parenting in the Black group (Pachter *et al*, 2006).

Patterns of relationships within families will also be important in mediating the effects of parental mental illness. Medication for the parent's disorder can reduce parental responsiveness and affect the parent–child relationship. High levels of criticism from a parent towards a child negatively impacts on the child's development and self-esteem, and the association between depression and other problems in the children of mothers with depression is, at least in part, related to the mother's increased levels of criticism of the child, rather than, for example, the child internalising the mother's own negative cognitions about herself (Jaenicke *et al*, 1987). Generally, it is the quality of the parent–child relationship and the quality of parenting, rather than the parental illness *per se*, that affects the child's development (Johnson *et al*, 2001). It has also been noted that coping styles differ in families where a parent has a mental illness, compared with those where the parents are well. Parents with depression and their children are more likely than well parents to use maladaptive, avoidance strategies such as self-blame, wishful thinking, not talking about problems, and worrying, and are less likely to seek external support (Cogan *et al*, 2004). Children who used strategies that are aimed at accepting or adapting to the stress of living with a parent with depression were less anxious, depressed or aggressive (Langrock *et al*, 2002).

Solantaus-Simula *et al* (2002) found that children had different ways of coping with parental low mood. They described four patterns of response – active empathy, emotional overinvolvement, indifference, and avoidance. These patterns were not related to the severity of the parental illness, and emotional overinvolvement and avoidance styles were found to be associated with more depressive and externalising symptoms in the children.

The gender of the child also exerts an influence. Rutter & Quinton (1984) found that boys of parents with a mental illness were more likely to develop conduct disorders, and that girls required longer periods of exposure before developing any problems. Children of the same gender as the ill parent appear to be at greatest risk (Goodyer *et al*, 1993).

As can be seen, the links mediating parental mental illness and child development are multifactorial, interactive and will operate differently at different stages of development. In a study examining the timing of maternal depressive symptoms and the effect on the child, McLean *et al* (2006) showed that both a history of maternal depression when the child was 2–4 months old and concurrent depression (when the child was 30–33 months old) affected (negatively) the child safety and child development practices of the mother when the child was 30–33 months. However, concurrent depressive symptoms had a stronger influence on child safety and child development practices as well as on harsh disciplinary practice at 30–33 months. In another study, remission of maternal depression was found to have a positive effect on both mothers and their children, with reduced rates of diagnoses and a reduced number of symptoms in the children. For those mothers, in this longitudinal study, who continued to have depression, there was an increase in the number of children who acquired a diagnosis (Weissman *et al*, 2006*b*). However, Cox *et al*, (1991) demonstrated that improvement in the mental state of mothers with depression did not necessarily lead to improvement in the child or in the parenting, suggesting that initiating mechanisms for child problems may not necessarily be the same as those that maintain difficulties.

## Resilience and protective factors

The relationships between parents with SMI and their children are generally good (Stallard *et al*, 2004), but children's ability to cope with their parents' mental illness will vary (Anthony, 1976). Good adaptation is associated with several factors: an older age when the parent becomes ill; an easier temperament and therefore an ability to form positive friendships; a higher IQ; parental illness characterised by an episodic course with good functioning between episodes; a supportive and positive relationship with other adults; and good achievements outside the home, for example at school or in sport (Rutter, 1988). Parent factors are also important. Goodman (1987) found that a better outcome for children of mothers with schizophrenia was associated with less severe maternal illness, an older age of the mother, higher levels of maternal education and maternal IQ, a history of the mother working, and the presence of another adult in the home. Therefore, despite the increased risk of childhood psychiatric disorders in children of mentally ill parents, individual and family circumstances will affect outcome, and therefore context is important. Parenting practice, rather than diagnosis, is often the most important factor in healthy child development.

In addition, practical arrangements, for example those involving service provision, can have a dramatic influence on promoting good outcome. Zankowski (1987) demonstrated that the most common reason women withdraw from their substance misuse treatment programme is a lack of child care arrangements. Compliance with these programmes is also better when child care is made available. Treatment programmes that consider the needs of the mother as a parent (in addition to her needs as a patient), such as psychoeducational approaches (Anderson *et al*, 1980; Falloon, 2000), may help children to develop protective mechanisms, and parents to avoid negatively affecting their children's development.

The needs of children with mentally ill parents include consideration of their needs as carers. Young carers are those who take on responsibilities for looking after their siblings and parents who are mentally ill. This can restrict their life experiences, for example educationally and socially, leading to isolation and lost opportunities. Services for young carers can address some of these difficulties by offering information and emotional support, as well as access to leisure activities and respite from the responsibilities of caring for their families.

## Learning from the experiences of children and families

Service providers for adults with mental illness rarely consider children. In one study, only 20% of case notes recorded the presence of children of their adult patients, and did not record their current circumstance (DeChillo *et al*, 1987). The complexity of the families' needs means that it is unlikely that one service alone will be able to address all of these needs, and there are likely to be competing priorities in different services. Parents complain that there is no service or plan to support their parenting (Dearden & Becker, 2000), and children feel ignored and left out. A young carer's project developed ten messages that children of mentally ill parents wanted conveyed to the professionals looking after their parents (*Keeping The Family In Mind*; Barnardo's, 2004). These included the need to receive information about mental illness generally and their parents' condition in particular; to be listened to, as they knew about their parents and the early signs of illness and relapse; to be relieved of guilt, as they commonly thought that they were to blame for their parents' illnesses; and to have a contact person with whom they could raise concerns. Many children also express concerns that they might catch their parents' illness.

A practical step that hospitals should take to help meet the needs of families is the provision of family visiting rooms that are child-friendly, and to formulate care plans that take into account the needs of children (Department of Health, 1999a).

What is required is a service, or services, that can address the parenting difficulties of mothers who are mentally ill, as well as their specific mental health needs. It would also need to address the emotional and behavioural problems of the children, while boosting the resilience and coping strategies of both parents and children. Such a service might begin to reduce the short- and longer-term effects of parental mental illness on children.

# 5 The development of the CAN–M

## Katherine Hunt and Louise Howard

Over 60% of women with an SMI are mothers (McGrath *et al*, 1999; Howard *et al*, 2001) and therefore an instrument that can assess their particular needs will be widely used. The CAN–M therefore includes examining needs in the area of violence and abuse; parenting and caring responsibilities; social and economic health; physical health; ethnicity and culture; substance misuse; and risk assessment. The instrument has also been developed to be used in as many service settings as possible, including acute psychiatric wards, mother and baby units, maternity and antenatal services, community mental health teams, social services and day centres.

## Four principles underlying the development of CAN–M

The overall format of the CAN was preserved in the development of the CAN–M and a number of the domains remain the same. The format, wording and particular emphasis of specific questions has been modified, however, to address the specific needs of pregnant women and mothers with SMI. The format of the CAN–M was based on four underlying principles:

1. Pregnant women and mothers with mental health problems have basic needs like everybody else, along with specific needs associated with their condition.
2. The primary aim of the instrument is to identify rather than describe in detail each need; once a need is identified, a more specialist assessment can be conducted.
3. A needs assessment should be suitable for use by a wide range of professionals, so that it can be applied in routine clinical practice.
4. Needs are subjective and therefore the service user and professionals' points of view should be recorded separately.

## Identification of new CAN–M need domains

### Method

We developed the new CAN–M need domains by, first, inviting service users and staff from in-patient and community mental health services to take part in individual interviews to discuss need domains that they felt were important in the context of developing an instrument to measure the needs of mothers with SMI. Inclusion criteria for service users were SMI and having children 16 years or younger, or a current pregnancy. Severe mental illness was defined by using the Threshold Assessment Grid (TAG; Slade *et al*, 2000), which is a validated method of identifying people with severe mental health problems (using a cut-off of 5 or more). The TAG consists of seven domains covering intentional self-harm, unintentional self-harm, risk from others, risk to others, survival (basic amenities, resources or living skills), psychological problems and social problems, which are graded according to severity. Women were excluded if they were deemed too ill by their consultant or had learning disabilities. Inclusion criteria for staff were experience in working with women with SMI who had been pregnant or had children aged 16 years or younger.

Service users were asked to provide comments to open questions regarding the needs of pregnant women and mothers with SMI, and to indicate which needs on a list of 35 health, social and psychological needs were most relevant for this particular group. This list comprised the 22 original CAN needs, and a further 13 needs identified by the researcher and the steering group committee as being potentially important to this group of service users. Women were also asked to name any other needs they felt were important and should be included. Similarly, mental health professionals from in-patient and community teams were individually interviewed and asked which domains they felt should be included. A thematic analysis was undertaken to identify the needs that received the greatest endorsement during interviews.

## Results

Semi-structured interviews took place with 13 service users (87% response rate) who had a mean TAG score of 10.3 (s.d.=2.3) and 19 staff members (100% response rate) recruited from a range of in-patient and out-patient community sites. Socio-demographic characteristics of the service users and staff are provided in Table 1. The majority of staff members were mental health nurses (12 (63%)), but 3 (16%) were social workers, and 1 psychiatrist, 1 psychologist, 1 occupational therapist and 1 nursing assistant were also interviewed.

A thematic analysis resulted in the identification of three new domains not previously included in CAN variants; *Pregnancy care*, *Sleep* and *Violence and abuse*, and three significantly modified CAN domains (*Safety to child/children and others*, *Practical demands of childcare* and *Emotional demands of childcare*).

Significant differences were identified between the service user and staff groups in terms of the endorsement of these specific needs. Service users suggested a domain of *Violence and abuse* significantly more often than the staff ($\chi^2$=4.57, P=0.03), and the staff suggested a domain of *Safety to child/children and others* significantly more often than the service users ($\chi^2$=4.98, P=0.03) (Table 2).

**Table 1** Service user and staff demographics

|  | Service user | Staff |
|---|---|---|
| Age, years: mean (s.d.) | 31.5 (10.2) | 37.4 (5.6) |
| Marital status, *n* (%) |  |  |
| Single | 8 (62) |  |
| Cohabiting/married | 3 (24) |  |
| Separated | 2 (15) |  |
| Recruitment, *n* (%) |  |  |
| Mother and baby unit | 5 (38) | 6 (32) |
| In-patient ward | 5 (38) | 6 (32) |
| Community out-patients | 3 (24) | 7 (36) |

**Table 2**  Interview theme frequencies with staff and service users

|  | Pregnancy care % | Sleep % | Violence and abuse % | Safety to child/ children and others % | Practical demands of childcare % | Emotional demands of childcare % |
|---|---|---|---|---|---|---|
| Staff | 58 | 42 | 37* | 53* | 63 | 53 |
| Service user | 38 | 46 | 77* | 15* | 38 | 54 |

*Statistically significant at $P=0.05$.

# Themes discussed in the interviews

Six new domains of *Pregnancy care, Sleep, Violence and abuse, Safety to child/children and others, Practical demands of childcare, Emotional demands of childcare* were included in the first draft of the CAN–M. Examples of the types of issues explored in the interviews are presented below. Two additional issues to arise from the interviews, stigma and discrimination and improving services for mothers with SMI, have also been presented below. Although neither of these issues are (strictly speaking) needs, they are relevant issues to service users and professionals working in this area, and therefore are discussed here for readers.

## Pregnancy care (domain 7)

Service users reported a number of physical problems relating to pregnancy and/or after the birth during the semi-structured interviews, including anaemia during pregnancy, premature birth, bleeding after birth, the loss of menstruation related to the post-partum period and medication, and the inability to produce sufficient milk following a stressful pregnancy. Staff also said that close monitoring was crucial for this group of women, as pregnant women with mental illness do not always engage with antenatal services. Poor attendance for antenatal care by women with mental illness has been reported in several studies (Wrede *et al*, 1980; Goodman & Emory, 1992; Miller & Finnerty, 1996). We have also reported that doctors are less likely to record routine aspects of antenatal care, for example smoking and alcohol consumption in women with psychotic disorders, even though these women are more likely to smoke and have substance misuse problems compared with matched controls (Howard *et al*, 2003a).

## Sleep (domain 8)

Many of the mothers reported experiencing sleep problems and required medication to help with sleep. Staff also spoke about the importance of having someone to share child night-time responsibilities as a means of helping mothers to receive sufficient sleep to be able to function the next day.

## Violence and abuse (domain 18)

Several service users described experiencing a traumatic childhood and growing up in children's homes or in families with social services involvement. Mothers also described more recent experiences of domestic violence, rape and financial exploitation. One woman described being wary of all men, including male professionals. Staff seemed to underestimate the high prevalence of violence and abuse experienced by service users, as they were significantly less likely to suggest this domain compared with service users. The failure of mental health care professionals to recognise the incidence of violence and abuse has also been reported in other studies (Read *et al*, 2005). However, staff indicated that asylum seekers often have traumatic experiences that need to be acknowledged and addressed.

## *Safety to child/children and others (domain 13)*

Staff said that safety to children was a very important area of need for mothers with SMI and that this required continuous assessment and monitoring. It was thought, however, that a mother and child should only be separated in very high-risk situations. One staff member spoke about her experience of caring for a mother who had attempted to murder her child and the ongoing grief that she experienced as a result of her thoughts. Safety issues were significantly less likely to be highlighted by the service users, possibly reflecting fear that disclosing problems in this area could lead to a loss of custody. Fear of custody loss has been reported as a central issue in the lives of these mothers (Krumm & Becker, 2006).

## *Practical demands of childcare (domain 19)*

Several service users described receiving inadequate information and training around the practical demands of childcare, such as nappy changing and discipline. Mothers described the importance of having a partner or family to help out with the demands of childcare, while another woman said that her parenting abilities were constantly being underestimated by professionals. Staff said that it was important to know exactly who would step in and perform the practical demands of childcare if there was a relapse, and that the normalisation and acknowledgement of parenting difficulties can often help to relieve some of the distress and anxiety experienced by the mothers.

## *Emotional demands of childcare (domain 20)*

One service user said that she had gone through a stage where she had rejected her new role of motherhood and did not want any contact with her baby. Another mother spoke of the importance of being well so that she could be around to protect her children, who she viewed as being vulnerable due to her mental illness. Staff spoke about the importance of allowing mothers to see their children during relapse to maintain an emotional connection, and the importance of mothers seeing a specialist if attachment problems arise.

## *Stigma and discrimination*

Stigma and discrimination were frequently discussed in the interviews. Several of the service users indicated that society was responsible for making them feel inferior and ignored. One mother said that people seem to 'treat you like a child' if you have a mental illness, and that people often make too many assumptions about patients' level of dangerousness. Another mother said 'People believe that everyone with a mental illness is capable of killing'. Healthcare professionals also felt that society required psychoeducation about women with mental illness to prevent stigma. Another member of staff recommended that mothers with mental illness be encouraged to use their own personal experiences to inform and empower others in similar situations. Many studies have found that women report negative reactions from others to pregnancy and motherhood (Savvidou *et al*, 2003; Diaz-Caneja & Johnson, 2004). Women talk about feeling continually monitored and suspected of abusing their children (Nicholson *et al*, 1998a). This perception of stigma may prevent women from seeking or receiving parenting support.

*Service provision*

Service users and staff believed that there was a need for improved services for pregnant women and mothers with SMI. Service users reported that it took an unacceptable length of time to get help from the National Health Service, as well as there being a lack of consistency with care. Many staff spoke of the long-standing communication difficulties between adult mental health services and social services, as well as the confusion that existed over who was taking the lead role in caring for these families. There was also support for the introduction of more preventative services and the importance of having clear care plans. The importance of introducing more flexibility and accessibility into the services, such as offering weekend and evening sessions was also emphasised.

## National survey to assess validity of individual domains of need

The first draft version of the CAN–M was sent to an advisory group to scrutinise the layout and wording. This group consisted of experts from a diverse range of professional backgrounds, including child psychiatry, psychology, occupational therapy, nursing and social work, as well as a service user. These comments resulted in minor changes to the instrument, and the creation of a new coversheet to ensure that child protection issues were adequately addressed in the instrument. The CAN–M therefore has acceptable face validity.

A survey of the second draft was then conducted to establish the content validity of the instrument. Service users and professional experts rated the proposed domains on a 5-point Likert scale of importance (ranging from 'Not at All' to 'Essential'). The service users were recruited from a range of in-patient and out-patient sites across south London, and the names and contact details of professional experts working with pregnant women and mothers with SMI were provided by the lead investigators on this project, members of the steering group committee and the advisory board. Participants were also invited to make suggestions for any other topics that they believed to be overlooked in the first draft. The statistical package STATA (version 9.1) was used to establish the content validity and consensual validity for the proposed domains in the CAN–M.

*Results*

The survey consisted of 63 (74%) service users, who had a mean TAG score of 8.1 (s.d.=2.9) and a mean age of 32.1 (s.d.=8.2), and 50 (68%) professional experts, details of whom are provided in Tables 3 and 4.

Content validity

The service user survey found that 24 out of the 25 domains had a mean importance score of 3 and above, thereby demonstrating that most rated these domains as being of at least 'Moderate importance' (Table 5). Four of the six new domains received a score of 4 and above, indicating that these needs were viewed as 'Very important' or 'Essential', with the *Pregnancy care* domain falling slightly below at 3.97. The highest scoring items were the *Practical demands of childcare* and *Safety to self* domains, while the lowest scoring domains were *Sexual health* and *Intimate relationships*.

Consensual validity

A parallel survey was conducted with 50 experts in order to establish consensual validity for the instrument. All 25 domains received an average importance score of 3 or above, indicating that the

**Table 3** Characteristics of service users participating in the study

| Status | n (%) |
|---|---|
| Marital | |
| Single | 32 (51) |
| Cohabiting/married | 24 (38) |
| Separated/divorced | 6 (10) |
| Widowed | 1 (2) |
| Patient | |
| In-patients | 32 (51) |
| Out-patients | 31 (49) |
| Motherhood | |
| Mother[a] | 53 (84) |
| Pregnant and mother[a] | 2 (3) |
| Pregnant, no other children | 8 (13) |

a. Of children 16 years and under.

**Table 4** Characteristics of professionals participating in the study

| Characteristic | n (%) |
|---|---|
| Profession | |
| Psychiatrists | 19 (38) |
| Nurses | 12 (24) |
| Social workers | 5 (10) |
| Psychologists | 4 (8) |
| Occupational therapists | 3 (6) |
| Midwife | 2 (4) |
| Other | 5 (10) |
| Area | |
| London | 30 (60) |
| England | 14 (28) |
| Wales/Scotland/Ireland | 4 (8) |
| Outside UK | 2 (4) |
| Years qualified: mean (s.d.) | 16.6 (8.8) |

experts viewed all listed domains as being at least 'Moderately important' (Table 6). The expert group also rated the five new CAN–M domains as having a score of 4 or above. The highest scoring domains were the *Safety to child/children and others* and *Safety to self* domains, while the lowest scoring items were, again, the *Sexual health* and *Intimate relationships* domains.

## Additional items of need

Service users and experts made suggestions for other areas of needs for inclusion in the new instrument. One additional area of need – *Language, culture and religion* – was identified by many respondents as

**Table 5**   Service users ratings of importance (scale 1–5)

| Domain | Mean (s.d.) |
| --- | --- |
| Accommodation | 3.92 (1.05) |
| Food | 3.9   (0.95) |
| Looking after the home | 3.83 (1.25) |
| Self-care | 3.6   (1.11) |
| Daytime activities | 4.37 (0.79) |
| General physical health | 4.22 (0.98) |
| Pregnancy care[a] | 3.97 (0.92) |
| Sleep[a] | 4.35 (0.67) |
| Psychotic symptoms | 4.49 (1.04) |
| Psychological distress | 4.44 (0.72) |
| Information | 4.51 (0.94) |
| Safety to self | 4.48 (0.95) |
| Safety to child/children and others[a] | 4.31 (0.95) |
| Substance misuse | 4.02 (0.99) |
| Company | 3.02 (1.27) |
| Intimate relationships | 2.92 (1.3) |
| Sexual health | 4.33 (0.8) |
| Violence and abuse[a] | 4.52 (0.74) |
| Practical demands of childcare[a] | 4.47 (0.69) |
| Emotional demands of childcare[a] | 3.45 (1.0) |
| Basic education | 3.53 (1.14) |
| Telephone | 3.48 (1.26) |
| Transport | 3.78 (1.16) |
| Budgeting | 4.22 (0.92) |
| Benefits | 4.22 (0.94) |

a. New CAN–M domain.

being particularly important. A domain covering the language, cultural and religious needs of women was therefore added to the final version of the instrument. This took the total number of need domains to 26.

## Assessment of reliability and concurrent validity

### *Method*

### Reliability

Following the development of the instrument described above, 36 subject-pairs consisting of a service user and a staff member were enrolled in a reliability study. Interviews were conducted 'live' by a lead rater and in the presence of a 'silent' second rater (time 1, T1). Permission to videotape interviews was sought from the service users and members of staff when a second rater was unable to attend. All tapes were destroyed following the completion of the evaluation. A total of six raters took part in the reliability study, each with varying professional skills and personal experience in the areas of research, service user

**Table 6** Staff ratings of importance (scale 1–5)

| Domain | Mean (s.d.) |
| --- | --- |
| Accommodation | 4.72 (0.54) |
| Food | 4.28 (0.76) |
| Looking after the home | 3.96 (0.78) |
| Self-care | 4.3  (0.68) |
| Daytime activities | 3.84 (0.87) |
| General physical health | 4.5  (0.71) |
| Pregnancy care[a] | 4.24 (0.96) |
| Sleep[a] | 4.18 (0.87) |
| Psychotic symptoms | 4.88 (0.39) |
| Psychological distress | 4.74 (0.49) |
| Information | 4.5  (0.68) |
| Safety to self | 4.92 (0.34) |
| Safety to child/children and others[a] | 4.98 (0.14) |
| Substance misuse | 4.62 (0.57) |
| Company | 3.9  (0.91) |
| Intimate relationships | 3.42 (1.03) |
| Sexual health | 3.1  (0.96) |
| Violence and abuse[a] | 4.54 (0.79) |
| Practical demands of childcare[a] | 4.86 (0.35) |
| Emotional demands of childcare[a] | 4.56 (0.61) |
| Basic education | 3.52 (0.95) |
| Telephone | 3.74 (0.94) |
| Transport | 3.58 (0.88) |
| Budgeting | 3.76 (0.82) |
| Benefits | 4.08 (0.94) |

a. New CAN–M domain.

experience, nursing, psychology and occupational therapy. No formal training was given to the raters, but they were given a brief explanation of the CAN–M coding algorithm. All raters rotated in their role as lead rater and silent rater. The level of agreement between the six raters provided an estimation of interrater reliability. All interviews performed at T1 were timed.

Test–retest reliability was also performed in order to give a measure of the instrument's stability over time. The rater who performed the interview at T1 was required to re-interview the same respondents at the second point in time (T2) without the presence of a second rater.

## Validity

Concurrent validity was assessed in order to determine the accuracy of the new CAN–M instrument. No widely accepted 'gold standard' instrument exists currently for the assessment of needs of pregnant women and mothers with severe mental health problems. Thus, in order to establish the concurrent validity of the CAN–M, the new instrument was compared with the two subscales of the Global Assessment of Functioning (GAF) (Endicott *et al*, 1976), which measure the severity of symptomology due to psychiatric symptoms (GAF–S), and the severity of disability (GAF–D). It was anticipated that the scores on the GAF–S and GAF–D would reflect an inverse relationship with the level of unmet needs identified by the

CAN–M. The concurrent validity was calculated first, by comparing the CAN–M summary scores (total number of needs) rated by staff with GAF subscales, and second, by comparing individually selected items from the CAN–M with the GAF subscales as identified by a recent study which examined factor loading of CAN needs (Korkeila *et al*, 2005). These items were selected with a view to providing a more representative measure of either symptomology or disability, and therefore giving a more meaningful estimate of concurrent validity.

## Statistical analysis

STATA version 9.0 was used for the analysis. A significance level of 5% was used. Non-parametric correlations (Spearman's *r*) were used for testing the concurrent validity. Concordance correlation coefficients were used for the interrater reliability and test–retest reliability analyses (Lin, 1989, Steichen & Cox, 2002) to measure absolute agreement. Absolute agreement is assessed, since this is generally the quantity of interest (typically mean levels of need would be compared between individuals and groups). Concordance correlations normally lie between 0 and 1, with values over 0.7 being generally regarded as acceptable and values over 0.9 as representing very good agreement. Paired *t*-tests were used to compare mean numbers of needs between users and staff, and between T1 and T2 values for the same user. Kappa coefficients were calculated for individual needs domains. In a few cases these could not be calculated because the responses were all at the ceiling or floor value. In addition, regression analyses were performed to investigate variation among individual raters (using the xtreg command in STATA, including patients as random effects and raters as fixed effects).

## *Results*

The socio-demographic characteristics of the 36 service users recruited for the reliability study are shown in Table 7. Twelve (33%) of the service users were recruited at mother and baby units, ten (28%) were recruited at community mental health team centres, nine (25%) were recruited at perinatal out-patient clinics, while the remaining five (14%) were recruited from in-patient wards. The mean age of the service users was 34.4 (s.d.=6.9) and the mean TAG score was 8.7 (s.d.=3.1). Two (6%) of the service users were pregnant with no children. Twenty-one (58%) had one child, nine (25%) had two children, and four (11%) had three or more children. Staff recruited included 17 (50%) nursing staff, 8 (24%) mental health workers, 4 (12%) health visitors, 2 (6%) social workers and 3 (9%) others (psychiatrist, counsellor, psychotherapist). Staff had known the service user for a mean 16.8 months (s.d.=25.3) with a minimum of 2 weeks and a maximum of 10 years. The time interval between T1 and T2 averaged 13 days (s.d.=6.7), and 87% of the participants interviewed at T1 were re-interviewed at T2. Young children were present at 13 (36%) T1 interviews. The mean duration of the interview at T1 for the service users was 23.3 minutes (s.d.=11.4) and the presence of children did not affect the interview duration ($t=-0.62$, mean difference$=-0.03$, 95% CI $-0.13$ to $0.07$, $P=0.54$). The mean duration for the T1 interview with staff was 18.3 minutes (s.d.=4.4). The mean total of needs (met and unmet) experienced by the service users at T1 was 7.69 (s.d.=4.31) as reported by the service users themselves, and 6.22 (s.d.=3.16) when reported by staff. The service users reported significantly more needs than the staff members ($t=3.67$, mean difference$=2.19$, 95% CI $0.97$ to $3.42$, $P<0.01$). The mean total number of needs reported by the service users did not differ depending on the presence or absence of young children in the interview room ($t=-0.57$, mean difference$=-0.28$, 95% CI $-3.45$ to $2.89$, $P=0.86$).

Analyses were also performed to identify the average number of unmet needs experienced by the service users at T1, that is, the average number of serious social or health problems experienced by the service users irrespective of the type or level of help received. Results showed that the mean total of unmet needs per service user at T1 was 5.51 (s.d.=4.39) and 3.42 (s.d.=3.01) as reported by the service user

**Table 7** Socio-demographic characteristics of service users in the evaluation study

|  | *n* (%) |
| --- | --- |
| Marital status |  |
| Single | 17 (47) |
| Cohabiting/married | 14 (39) |
| Separated/divorced | 4 (11) |
| Widowed | 1  (3) |
| Ethnicity |  |
| White | 16 (44) |
| Black | 13 (36) |
| Asian | 2  (6) |
| Other | 5 (14) |
| Age at leaving full-time education, years |  |
| 11 | 1  (3) |
| 14–15 | 10 (28) |
| 16–18 | 11 (31) |
| 19 and above | 8 (25) |
| Employment status |  |
| Medically retired | 15 (42) |
| Employed | 8 (22) |
| Unemployed | 11 (31) |
| Student | 1  (3) |
| Other | 1  (3) |
| Number of children aged ≤16 years |  |
| Pregnant with no children | 2  (6) |
| 1 | 21 (58) |
| 2 | 9 (25) |
| 3+ | 4 (11) |
| Custody of youngest child |  |
| Mother | 23 (68) |
| Father (if separated) | 3  (9) |
| Relatives | 5 (15) |
| Adopted | 3  (9) |
| Living with child? |  |
| Yes | 25 (74) |
| No | 9 (26) |
| Living with other adults? |  |
| No | 9 (25) |
| Spouse/partner | 12 (33) |
| Parents | 6 (17) |
| Unrelated others | 5 (14) |
| Child 16+ years old | 3  (8) |
| Other relatives | 1  (3) |
| Clinical diagnosis |  |
| Schizophrenia or other psychotic disorder | 11 (31) |
| Depressive disorder | 11 (31) |

**Table 7** (Continued)   Socio-demographic characteristics of service users in the evaluation study

|  | *n* (%) |
|---|---|
| Bipolar affective disorder | 8 (22) |
| Anxiety disorder | 3 (8) |
| Personality disorder | 1 (3) |
| Not known | 2 (6) |
| Service contact |  |
| 0–6 months | 6 (17) |
| 6–12 months | 9 (25) |
| 2–5 years | 4 (11) |
| >5 years | 17 (47) |
| Number of lifetime psychiatric admissions |  |
| No hospital admission | 8 (23) |
| 1 | 13 (37) |
| 2–4 | 8 (23) |
| 5 or more | 6 (17) |

and staff, respectively. A paired *t*-test showed that the service users reported significantly more unmet needs compared to the staff ($t=4.12$, mean difference$=2.55$, 95% CI 1.29 to 3.81, $P<0.001$), with the seven most common types of unmet need being psychological distress (in 51%), sleeping problems and budgeting (both 40%), an inability to preoccupy themselves during the day with appropriate daytime activities (in 37%), and an absence of information, feelings of social isolation and personal difficulties relating to either past or current experiences of violence and abuse (each 34%).

## Reliability

Concordance correlation coefficients between the total CAN–M summary scores of the two raters for total number of needs (interrater reliability) and at the two time points of T1 and T2 (test–retest reliability) were calculated. The concordance coefficients for the interrater analysis were 0.99 for the service user ratings and 0.95 for the staff ratings. For the test–retest reliability, the coefficients were 0.92 and 0.79 for the service users and staff respectively. The total number of needs (met and unmet) across the two time points did not differ significantly for either the service users ($t=1.61$, mean difference$=0.47$, 95% CI $-0.12$ to 1.06, $P=0.12$) or staff ($t=0.93$, mean difference$=0.44$, 95% CI $-0.54$ to 1.42, $P=0.36$), nor did the time between T1 and T2 differ significantly between the service users and staff ($t=-1.52$, mean difference$=-0.96$, 95% CI $-2.26$ to 0.35, $P=0.14$).

Results were also calculated using the total number of unmet needs as reported by the two raters. The results of the interrater analysis were 0.93 for the service users and 0.83 for the staff. The test–retest reliability coefficients were 0.91 and 0.85 for the service users and staff respectively. These results show that the CAN–M has excellent agreement, both between different raters and on different occasions, for identifying serious problems in pregnant women and mothers with SMI (Howard *et al*, 2007).

No systematic bias in rating styles was identified between the lead and silent raters in identifying needs in pregnant women and mothers with SMI (mean difference$=-0.03$, 95% CI $-1.33$ to 1.27 for the service users; mean difference$=-0.38$, 95% CI $-2.29$ to 1.54 for staff).

## Concurrent validity

The total summary scores for unmet needs were compared with the GAF–S and GAF–D. The mean GAF–S score was 60.8 (s.d.=13.5) and the mean GAF–D score was 59.8 (s.d.=15.0). The Spearman's *r* correlation coefficients were moderated with the GAF–S –0.36 (*P*=0.05) and was –0.52 with the GAF–D (*P*<0.01). These relationships were found to strengthen with: (a) the removal of the *General physical health* domain (as GAF–S assesses psychiatric symptomatology only) and the inclusion of CAN–M specific domains of *Safety to child/children and others* and *Sleep* (–0.62, *P*<0.001) and (b) domains associated with impairment (including the two new childcare domains, domains assessing abilities, such as buying and preparing meals (*Food*), keeping the house clean and tidy (*Looking after the home*), and using public transport (*Transport*) (as these were relevant to the GAF–D) (–0.44, *P*=0.01).

## Sections 2 and 3

Descriptive analyses were performed to examine the reported levels of support received by the service users from both informal supports, such as partner, friends and relatives (Section 2 of the CAN–M), and more formal supports, such as hospital staff and local services (Section 3a of the CAN–M) (Table 8). There were no significant differences between the service user and staff ratings in terms of whether or not support was received by the service users from informal sources, i.e. relatives and friends (McNemar test $\chi^2(1)=2.14$, *P*=0.14), though staff were often unsure about the level of help received by the user from their partner, friends and relatives to meet their needs. A significant difference was found between the staff and service user ratings in terms of whether or not support was received by local services (McNemar test $\chi^2(1)=9.67$, *P*=0.002). Service users and staff were also found to differ in terms of whether or not there was a perceived level of support needed from services in order to meet the service user's needs (McNemar test $\chi^2(1)=10.65$, *P*=0.002).

## Section 4

Both service users and staff were asked whether the service users received the right type of help to meet their needs (Section 4a) (Table 9). There was a significant difference between the user and staff ratings in regard to the appropriateness of the help received, with the service users being more likely to respond 'No' to this question (McNemar test $\chi^2(1)=4.3$, *P*=0.04).

**Table 8**  User and staff ratings on Sections 2 and 3

| Level of help | None n (%) | | Low help n (%) | | Moderate help n (%) | | High help n (%) | | Not known n (%) | |
|---|---|---|---|---|---|---|---|---|---|---|
| Section question | User | Staff | User | Staff | User | Staff | User | Staff | User | Staff |
| How much help does the person receive from partner, friends or relatives? (2) | 96 (36) | 69 (33) | 56 (21) | 57 (27) | 64 (24) | 27 (13) | 49 (18) | 29 (14) | 3 (1) | 30 (14) |
| How much help does the person receive from local services? (3a) | 119 (44) | 32 (15) | 50 (19) | 66 (31) | 54 (20) | 49 (23) | 43 (16) | 58 (28) | 2 (1) | 6 (3) |
| How much help does the person need from local services? (3b) | 29 (11) | 13 (6) | 40 (15) | 46 (22) | 87 (33) | 69 (33) | 94 (35) | 77 (37) | 18 (7) | 5 (2) |

**Table 9**    User and staff ratings on the right type of help

| Section question | Yes, *n* (%) | | No, *n* (%) | | Not known, *n* (%) | |
|---|---|---|---|---|---|---|
| | User | Staff | User | Staff | User | Staff |
| Does the person receive the right type of help? | 142 (53) | 140 (76) | 104 (39) | 58 (28) | 21 (8) | 12 (6) |

The service users were then asked an additional question in Section *4b* of the CAN–M which examined their overall levels of satisfaction in having their needs met. The results showed that 20% of the total number of needs identified by the service users themselves were rated as being appropriately met and the service users were satisfied with the overall levels of support received. In contrast, 39% of the needs identified were described as being unmet and the service users were dissatisfied with the help received.

# Conclusion

This chapter has described the development of the CAN–M and demonstrated that the CAN–M has a high level of reliability and validity. The results provided here also illustrate the importance of both service user and staff perspectives, as these are frequently significantly different.

# 6 Guidance on rating

## Katherine Hunt and Louise Howard

## Practical issues

The interviewer using the CAN–M should be a professional who has knowledge and experience of working with pregnant women and mothers with SMI. Formal training in the use of CAN–M is not necessary but certain challenges may be encountered when working with this particular population group, and we would therefore recommend that staff identify and explore these issues before using the CAN–M, either within service settings or during a training session. Interviewers should know how to interview people with impaired concentration and psychotic symptoms. It should also be noted that some service users might choose to have their babies or children with them when they attend a needs assessment; certain topics of discussion are not thought to be suitable for older children (e.g. needs relating to safety to self and abuse experiences) and therefore their presence is not recommended in the interview room. Similarly, family members and friends may also impact on the service user's ability to talk freely about their needs. Therefore a more accurate assessment of needs may be attained if they are not present.

When using the CAN–M, it is recommended that the session commence with a brief explanation of the duration and purpose of the interview. This explanation might take the form:

> 'This assessment asks a number of questions about areas that pregnant women and mothers can sometimes have difficulties with. There are 26 broad areas of need to cover, and some of them may not be relevant or applicable to you. Each question follows exactly the same format, asking if you have had any difficulties in the area during the past month. (If the CAN–M(R) or CAN–M (C) are being used, add "If you have experienced any difficulties in this area, I would then like to ask about any help you have been receiving, first from your partner, friends and realtives, then from the services. I will also be asking whether you feel that you are receiving the right type of help for your needs from services and whether you are satisfied with the help you have been receiving.") I will go through each question in turn and please let me know if there is anything you do not understand. As I said before, if there are any questions you would prefer not to answer, please say so and we can move on to the next question. Do you have any questions you would like to ask me before we start?'

The interviewer should also give some indication about how long the interview will take in total. A full assessment will usually take about 15–25 minutes to complete, and the short version around 5–10 minutes. The duration of the interview may vary, however, depending on the number of identified needs of the person being assessed. Each of the domains is self-contained and so breaks can be taken as required. The CAN–M domains are ordered in such as way as to leave the more personal questions to later in the interview, thereby allowing time for the respondent to feel more comfortable with the interview format.

Two different perspectives are assessed using the CAN–M: the user and the staff member. It is this view (not the view of the interviewer) that is recorded. The interviewee may be the service user or a member of staff (e.g. the care coordinator). If the service user is being interviewed, administration involves the interviewer going through the CAN–M, asking the service user about each domain in turn.

If a member of staff is the interviewee, this normally involves a member of staff completing the CAN–M him/herself. The user and staff views are recorded in separate columns to provide each person with the opportunity to express their own views on the needs of the user. There are no 'right' or 'wrong' answers. So, for example, the staff members should give their own views about service users' needs, rather than what they think the service users' views are.

The assessment procedure in each domain is identical. The suggested trigger questions, shown in italics, may be used to open discussions in each of the 26 domains. Additional questions should be asked with the goal of establishing whether the user has a need (currently met or unmet) in this domain.

---

If the needs domain is not applicable to the respondent,
    **rate 8 (not applicable)**, otherwise
if the respondent does not know or does not want to answer the question,
    **rate 9 (not known)**, otherwise
if a serious problem is present, irrespective of help given,
    **rate 2 (unmet need)**, otherwise
if there is no serious problem
    **rate 1 (met need)**, if this is because of help given, or
    **rate 0 (no need)**, if no help is given

---

# Rating algorithm

A rating algorithm can be used to identify whether needs are met or unmet. This applies to both the CAN–M (R) Section 1, CAN–M (C) Section 1 and the CAN–M (S) form. A more detailed description of scoring procedure can be found in Chapter 8.

# Specific rating issues in each need domain

On rating each of the 26 domains, there are some specific issues that have been found to require clarification.

## 1. Accommodation

This domain refers to the person's current housing situation in terms of how appropriate it is. If a person is currently in hospital and does not have an appropriate home to be discharged to, the needs rating is 1 (unmet need). However, if a person is in hospital and does have an appropriate home to be discharged to, the needs rating is 0 (no need). It is important to consider whether the home is appropriate for meeting the needs of both the mother and the child in this domain (i.e. whether the house is child safe).

## 2. Food

This domain refers to the person's ability to buy appropriate food (e.g. nutritional content, quantity, etc.) and whether she has the skills to prepare simple meals for both herself and, if applicable, for her child or children. If the person is an in-patient, however, this option may not be available, in which case scores should be made according to the appropriateness of the food provided by the service (either a met or unmet need).

## 3. *Looking after the home*

This domain refers to the person's ability to keep her living space in an adequate level of cleanliness, irrespective of whether it is an in-patient bedroom, supported housing or a rented flat. If the person is homeless, the respondent may be able to state whether they believe it would be a problem if she had a home; if not, a rating of 9 (not known) is given. If the service user displays obsessive–compulsive tendencies towards house cleaning, rate this domain as no needs (0), but rate the user as having unmet needs (2) in domain 10 (*Psychological distress*).

## 4. *Self-care*

This domain refers to a person's ability to perform basic self-care activities, in terms of both bodily cleanliness and clothing. It does not include unusual, eccentric or bizarre appearance.

## 5. *Daytime activities*

This domain refers to whether the person has enough to do during the day and whether she can occupy herself with suitable activities. If the primary problem is loneliness and isolation, rather than inactivity and boredom, then this should be rated under the domain of *Company*.

## 6. *General physical health*

This domain refers to the general physical health of the service user and it excludes all physical problems relating to pregnancy and birth. General disabilities and medication side-effects also need to be considered in this domain.

## 7. *Pregnancy care*

This domain refers to the physical health of the service user during her pregnancy and after the birth. If a pregnant service user discloses no significant physical health problems but says she is attending regular antenatal appointments for routine monitoring, rate the need as being met (1). Alternatively, if a pregnant service user has disclosed untreated physical complications related to the pregnancy or fails to attend antenatal appointments, the need is rated as unmet (2). This domain may be rated as not applicable (8) if the woman is not pregnant, if she has not given birth recently, or if she does not attribute any current health problems to a pregnancy or birth.

## 8. *Sleep*

This domain refers to difficulties with sleep, whether it is related to general insomnia, night-time childcare responsibilities, or sleeping difficulties due to late pregnancy. Sleeping aids may be used as a type of help and this can refer to a large range of activities, including relaxation music, relaxation exercises, massage and drinking warm milk drinks before bedtime. Although severely disrupted sleep has been identified as the primary cause of an unmet need in the CAN–M, women who require excessive amounts of sleep (e.g. 12 hours per night) may also rate their sleep needs as unmet (2).

## 9. Psychotic symptoms

This domain refers to any psychotic symptoms experienced by the service user. It is necessary to enquire about any medications she may be taking (if not mentioned in the previous domain concerning general physical health) and what these medications are for.

## 10. Psychological distress

This domain refers to any distress, anxiety or depression of a moderate to severe degree, regardless of the cause. Distress could include adjustment difficulties, a sense of helplessness, or overwhelming feelings of guilt and loss.

## 11. Information

This domain refers to the quality and comprehensiveness of information received by the service user regarding their condition, care plan and their rights. Information relating to their child's care plan and any additional child protection plans also need to be considered here. Emphasising that the questioning refers to difficulties and help received in the past month only is important – information might have been received in the past and the person might therefore not currently need any help in this area (in which case, the domain should be scored as no need).

## 12. Safety to self

This domain refers to both intentional and unintentional acts of self-harming behaviour. The issue of safety from others, for example exploitation and abuse, are rated under domain 18 (*Violence and abuse*).

## 13. Safety to child/children and others

This domain refers to threatening and violent behaviour exhibited by the service user towards her children or others. This behaviour can be either intentional or unintentional. Acts of excessive physical discipline with children should also be considered in this domain. If the person has been violent in the past month, this domain is automatically scored as an unmet need (2), regardless of subsequent preventative or therapeutic interventions.

## 14. Substance misuse

This domain refers to problematic and harmful substance misuse. This covers a wide range of substances including alcohol, cannabis, and all illicit drugs (e.g. heroin, cocaine, LSD), and the over-consumption of prescribed medication. The lack of access to drugs, for example if the service user is an in-patient, might not detract from an underlying problem or need in this area.

## 15. Company

This domain refers to social contacts and the ability to initiate conversation and form relationships with other people. Some people may indicate a preference for their own company and may not seek out friendships or support, in which case the domain should be scored as 'no needs'.

## 16. Intimate relationships

This domain refers to close personal relationships such as with a boyfriend, partner or husband. Some people may indicate a lack of interest in forming intimate relationships, in which case the domain should be scored as 'no needs'. Sensitivity may be necessary is exploring this and the next five domains.

## 17. Sexual health

This domain refers to difficulties the service user may be having with their sex lives and sexual functioning. This would include problems relating to a decreased libido, sexual problems during pregnancy or after the birth, contraception, safe sex practices and other family planning issues.

## 18. Violence and abuse

This domain assesses the presence of both past and current acts of violence and abuse against the service user. If she has disclosed current violence or abuse, or is extremely vulnerable to future violence and abuse, rate the individual as having unmet needs (2). Alternatively, if the service user has disclosed an experience of abuse and is receiving help for this issue either through informal sources such as family or friends, or formal sources such as a counsellor, rate the person as having met needs (1). If the service user has no experience of abuse or if she has developed adequate coping skills to deal with this experience and knows how to protect herself from future abuse, rate the person as having no needs (0).

## 19. Practical demands of childcare

This domain refers to difficulties the user may be having with the practical demands of looking after a child. This can be particularly relevant if the person is an in-patient, undergoing a parenting assessment, or if social services are involved. This can be perceived as a sensitive domain for some women and there may be fears that disclosure of parenting difficulties may automatically lead to child removal. This domain includes whether the mother is capable of providing adequate supervision, as well as setting boundaries and effective discipline. For younger children, it would also include activities such as assistance with eating meals, bathing, and brushing teeth. If the service user is pregnant with no other children or has no contact with her children (i.e. due to adoption), this domain should be rated as not applicable (8).

## 20. Emotional demands of childcare

This domain refers to difficulties the service user may be having in feeling emotionally close to her child. This can be perceived as a sensitive domain for some mothers. The domain includes whether the mother is capable of expressing appropriate affection and warmth towards her child, and whether the mother expresses hostility or over-protectiveness. If the service user has no contact with her child (e.g. due to adoption), then the domain should be rated as not applicable (8).

## 21. Basic education

This domain refers to basic education only, such as the ability to read a shop name, write a simple letter and count change received. Service users who do not have English as their primary language, but who attained a good level of schooling in a different country and who (through an interpreter) report no difficulties in reading, writing and counting in their primary language should receive a score of no needs (0). Their difficulties with the English language, however, should be coded in domain 26 (*Language, culture and religion*).

## 22. Telephone

This domain refers to the difficulties the person might have in getting access to or using the telephone. In-patients who have access to a ward telephone but who say they experience a lack of privacy should have their needs rated as unmet (2).

## 23. Transport

This domain refers to any difficulties the person may be having in accessing transport facilities or practical difficulties associated with the use of public transport, such as reading timetables, social phobia, physical health or childcare reasons.

## 24. Budgeting

This domain refers to the difficulties a person might be having in managing her money and whether she has the basic skills to pay for bills, food, clothes, etc. If the service user is an in-patient, ask if she has a nominated trusted person who is looking after her finances and paying bills while she is in hospital. If this is the case, rate the need as being met (1). Alternatively, if the user is in serious debt or has no one to oversee her finances while in hospital, rate the need as unmet (2).

## 25. Benefits

This domain refers to the difficulties a person might have with receiving the appropriate amount of benefits, according to her personal, social and family situation. If the user indicates that she is not sure whether she is getting the full benefit, rate the need as unmet (2).

## 26. Language, culture and religion

This domain refers to the difficulties a person might experience in having her specific language, cultural or religious needs met while being an in-patient or living with the community. This can include difficulties with speaking the main language in her area, access to certain clothes, requiring specific religious or cultural diets, and being provided with the opportunities to practice her faith.

# 7 Scoring the CAN–M

## Katherine Hunt and Louise Howard

There are three versions of the CAN–M: CAN–M (C), CAN–M (R) and CAN–M (S). The versions differ on the purpose of the interview, the amount of detail recorded, and the time taken to complete the assessment. The CAN–M (C), CAN–M (R) and CAN–M (S) are located in Appendices 2, 3 and 4 respectively, with summary score sheets for CAN–M (C) and CAN–M (R) in Appendices 5 and 6 respectively. Instructions for recording these different versions are presented below.

## Scoring the CAN–M (C)

The CAN–M (C) is a semi-structured interview schedule intended for clinical use which provides information on the service user's met and unmet needs. The CAN–M (C) has four sections for each domain, and is completed separately by the staff and the service user. The purpose of Section 1 is twofold: first, to assess whether there is a need in the domain, and whether effective help has already being given, and second, to decide whether further questions about this domain are necessary. Section 2 assesses the amount of help received from informal sources (friends, relatives, etc.). Section 3 assesses the amount of help given by and needed from formal services. For all ratings, anchor points and rating guidelines are provided. Section 4 records the service user's perceptions about the domain, and the staff care plan.

The CAN–M (C) assesses 26 domains of health and social needs which are described in detail in Chapter 6. Questions are asked about each domain, to identify:

(a)   whether a need or problem is present in the domain
(b)   whether the need is met or unmet. A need is met if there is currently not a problem in the domain, but a problem would exist if it were not for the help provided (i.e. the service user is getting effective help). A need is unmet if there is currently a problem in the domain (whether or not any help is currently being provided)
(c)   how much help the service user is currently receiving from informal (friends, relatives, etc.) or formal sources, and how much help she needs
(d)   the service user's views about her needs.

Space is also provided for staff to record the care plan relevant to this domain. At the end of an assessment, therefore, it is possible to say how many needs the service user has from these 26 domains, what help she is currently receiving and what help is needed, and her perspective about the difficulties.

*Note:* A CAN–M (C) assessment by itself may not be sufficient, so the care plan may include a need for further assessment.

Each CAN–M (C) can be used to record the perceptions of the staff and the service user. To avoid bulky notes, 1-page summary sheets are provided in Appendix 5, which are suitable for case notes.

*Section 1*

This section introduces the area of need to the respondent and is used to open a focused discussion on the topic. It aims to identify the presence or absence of need by asking the respondent if she has any problems in a particular area. Before deciding on a needs rating, it is important to establish whether a service user has no needs because of the benefits she is receiving from an effective intervention, or because she actually has no problems in this area of her life. Failure to clarify this matter can result in an underrating of needs. The anchor points (examples provided alongside each rating option) should be used *only* to guide the interviewer's rating response, as not all possible scenarios can be covered in the limited space provided. Clinical judgement may therefore be required in selecting the most appropriate response for each user. Five possible scoring options are available for Section 1. Each service user and staff score needs to be written in the columns provided along the right-hand side of every page.

## Rating a domain as no need (a score of 0)

A rating of 'no need' (0) indicates that the service user does not experience any current problems or difficulties for this particular area, nor does she receive any interventions. Careful attention must be paid to recording only needs that have been present in the past month, especially as some users may have experienced past serious difficulties in any one domain. An example here might be a long-term service user who had past difficulties understanding her condition, care plan and rights, but has since received sufficient information and has not required any additional information for the past 12 months.

## Rating a domain as met need (a score of 1)

A rating of a met need (1) would indicate that the service user does currently experience some difficulties in a particular area, but that effective intervention is reducing the extent of the problem. An example here might be the recent introduction of domestic help to a service user who struggles to keep the home clean and tidy.

## Rating a domain as unmet need (a score of 2)

A rating of an unmet need (2) would indicate that the service user is experiencing current difficulties in that particular domain. These difficulties should be of a serious or severe nature. It is important to note that a service user may be in receipt of some type of intervention but may still have unmet needs in this area, especially if she views the intervention as being ineffective or unnecessary in the management of her care. An example here might be the prescription of antidepressants for a service user who claims that the medication has done nothing to reduce her depression or distress.

## Rating domain as not applicable (a score of 8)

A needs rating of not applicable (8) is available for three CAN–M domains, these being *Pregnancy care* (domain 8), *Practical demands of childcare* (domain 19) and *Emotional demands of childcare* (domain 20). The *Pregnancy care* domain is rated as not applicable when the service user has not given birth in the past 12 months, and does not attribute any ongoing physical complications to a pregnancy or birth (irrespective of the time that has lapsed since the last birth). Domains 19 and 20 are rated as not applicable only if the user has no contact with the child owing to permanent removal such as adoption.

## Rating domain as not known (a score of 9)

A rating of not known (9) can be scored when the respondent either does not know the answer to a question (that is, the person cannot decide on how to answer a question), or does not wish to disclose information pertaining to any difficulties they might be experiencing. Staff members may also score not known (9) if they have not previously discussed a particular area of need with the user and so are unaware of the presence or absence of a need. A common example here would be discussing sexual health topics such as whether she is satisfied in her sexual relationship.

## *Section 2*

Section 2 is only completed when the respondent states that a need (met or unmet) exists. The section assesses the level of help provided to the service user by informal sources of support such as her partner, friends or relatives. In particular, the respondent is asked to indicate how helpful the service user's informal supports have been in the past month in meeting her personal needs. For example, if the service user states that she is receiving constant support and supervision (high level) from her husband in an attempt to alleviate her depression, but feels that this support is unhelpful or even making matters worse, then the perceived level of help should be rated as none (0). If the respondent has mentioned the names of a particular partner, friend or relative, then the interviewer should personalise the question, but not exclude other people who may be providing support. It is important to note that this section only taps into the level of help received by the service user from informal supports, not the level of help *needed*. Section 2 of the CAN–M (C) is scored according to a sliding scale of help received, with the addition of a 'not known' option.

| | |
|---|---|
| **0 = None** | No help received from informal supports for this area of need |
| **1 = Low help** | The respondent perceives any support in this areas as being a little helpful |
| **2 = Moderate help** | The respondent perceives any support in this areas as being moderately helpful |
| **3 = High help** | The respondent perceives any support in this areas as being very helpful |
| **9 = Not known** | The respondent is unable to say how helpful informal supports have been in meeting needs |

## *Section 3*

Section 3 is completed only if a need (met or unmet) has been previously identified in Section 1. This section assesses the level of help provided by local services such as mental health workers, general practitioners, health visitors or social workers. In particular, the respondent is asked to indicate how helpful the local services have been in the past month in meeting her personal needs. For example, if the service user has received details of domestic violence programmes in the past month (low help), but states that this help has done nothing to meet her needs, then the perceived level of help needs to be rated as none (0). It is important to note that unlike Section 2, this section assesses both *received* help (Section 3a) and help that is *needed* by local services (Section 3b). This section has the same rating options as Section 2.

| | |
|---|---|
| **0 = None** | No help received from local services for this area of need |
| **1 = Low help** | The respondent perceives any support in this areas as being a little helpful |

| | |
|---|---|
| **2 = Moderate help** | The respondent perceives any support in this areas as being moderately helpful |
| **3 = High help** | The respondent perceives any support in this areas as being very helpful |
| **9 = Not known** | The respondent is unable to say how helpful local services have been in meeting needs |

## Section 4

The purpose of this section is twofold:

1.    To record any information given by the service user that is not captured by the ratings, such as what help she would like in the future. This is only to be completed during the service user interview.

2.    To write action plans, which record what will be done (e.g. further assessment, specified intervention), who will do it and when the plan will be reviewed. This is completed by the member of staff.

CAN–M (C) ratings can be recorded directly in the boxes on the form. Alternatively, three summary score sheets are given in Appendix 5, which can be used to record an assessment. These summary sheets are shorter and more suitable for case notes than a complete CAN–M (C). The CAN–M (C) complete assessment summary sheet records a staff and a service user assessment of need, and the staff and service user assessment summary sheets record individual assessments by the staff or the service user. Each summary sheet allows the recording of summary variables: total number of met (needs rating 1) and unmet (needs rating 2) needs, the total number of needs (i.e. the sum of met and unmet needs), the total level of help received from informal and formal sources, and the total level of help needed from formal sources. In adding up these totals, always count an 8 (not applicable) or a 9 (not known) as 0. A record of the views of the service user and any action plans will also need to be kept, for example on the back of the summary score sheet.

Information from the CAN–M (C) can be used for at least two purposes:

(a)    Data can be used at the level of the individual user, by providing a baseline measure of level of need, or for charting changes over time. For example, one approach would be to use the CAN–M (C) routinely in initial assessments of new service users who are pregnant or are mothers, to identify the range of domains in which they are likely to require further assessment and (possibly) help or treatment.

(b)    Data can be used for auditing and developing an individual service. For example, to investigate:

(i)   the impact on needs of providing an intervention for pregnant women or mothers with SMI, by looking at changes across this group

(ii)  case-load dependency for different care coordinators

(iii) whether enough service users have unmet needs in certain domains to make it worthwhile for a community mental health team to provide relevant interventions (e.g. a welfare benefits adviser).

## Scoring the CAN–M (R)

The CAN–M (R) is a semi-structured interview schedule which provides information on the user's met and unmet needs. The CAN–M (R) has four sections for each domain, and is completed separately by the staff and the service user. The purpose of Section 1 is twofold: first, to assess whether there is a need in the domain, and whether effective help has already been given, and second, to decide whether further questions about this domain are necessary. Section 2 assesses the amount of help received from informal sources (friends, relatives, etc.). Section 3 assesses the amount of help given by and needed from formal services. For all ratings, anchor points and rating guidelines are provided. Section 4 records whether service users are getting the right type of help for their problems and, in the service user interview only, whether they are satisfied with the amount of help that they are receiving. It therefore differs from the CAN–M (C) in that it assesses satisfaction and does not record qualitative information on the service user's perspective of the action plan.

## *Section 1*

This section introduces the area of need to the respondent and is used to open a focused discussion on the topic. It aims to identify the presence or absence of need by asking the respondent if she has any problems in a particular area. Before deciding on a needs rating, it is important to establish whether a service user has no needs because of the benefits she is receiving from an effective intervention, or because she actually has no problems in this area of her life. Failure to clarify this matter can result in an underrating of needs. The anchor points (examples provided alongside each rating option) should be used *only* to guide the interviewer's rating response, as not all possible scenarios can be covered in the limited space provided. Clinical judgement may therefore be required in selecting the most appropriate response for each user. Five possible scoring options are available for Section 1. Each service user and staff score needs to be written in the columns provided along the right-hand side of every page.

### Rating a domain as no need (a score of 0)

A rating of 'no need' (0) indicates that the service user does not experience any current problems or difficulties for this particular area, nor does she receive any interventions. Careful attention must be paid to recording only needs that have been present in the past month, especially as some service users may have experienced past serious difficulties in any one domain. An example here might be a long-term service user who had past difficulties understanding her condition, care plan and rights, but has since received sufficient information and has not required any additional information for the past 12 months.

### Rating a domain as met need (a score of 1)

A rating of a met need (1) would indicate that the service user does currently experience some difficulties in a particular area, but that effective intervention is reducing the extent of the problem. An example here might be the recent introduction of domestic help to a service user who struggles to keep the home clean and tidy.

### Rating a domain as unmet need (a score of 2)

A rating of an unmet need (2) would indicate that the service user is experiencing current difficulties in that particular domain. These difficulties should be of a serious or severe nature. It is important to note that a service user may be in receipt of some type of intervention but may still have unmet needs in this area, especially if she views the intervention as being ineffective or unnecessary in the management of her care. An example here might be the prescription of antidepressants for a service user who claims that the medication has done nothing to reduce her depression or distress.

## Rating domain as not applicable (a score of 8)

A needs rating of not applicable (8) is available for three CAN–M domains, these being *Pregnancy care* (domain 8), *Practical demands of childcare* (domain 19) and *Emotional demands of childcare* (domain 20). The *Pregnancy care* domain is rated as not applicable when the service user has not given birth in the past 12 months and does not attribute any ongoing physical complications to a pregnancy or birth (irrespective of the time that has lapsed since birth). Domains 19 and 20 are rated as not applicable if the service user has no contact with the child owing to permanent removal such as adoption.

## Rating domain as not known (a score of 9)

A rating of not known (9) can be scored when the respondent either does not know the answer to a question (that is, the person cannot decide on how to answer a question), or does not wish to disclose information pertaining to any difficulties they might be experiencing. Staff members may also score not known (9) if they have not previously discussed a particular area of need with the service user and so are unaware of the presence or absence of a need.

## Section 2

Section 2 is only completed when the respondent states that a need (met or unmet) exists. The section assesses the level of help provided to the service user by informal sources of support such as her partner, friends or relatives. In particular, the respondent is asked to indicate how helpful the service user's informal supports have been in the past month in meeting her personal needs. For example, if the service user states that she is receiving constant support and supervision (high level) from her husband in an attempt to alleviate her depression, but feels that this support is unhelpful or even making matters worse, then the perceived level of help should be rated as none (0). If the respondent has mentioned the names of a particular partner, friend or relative, then the interviewer should personalise the question but not exclude other people who may be providing support. It is important to note that this section only taps into the level of help received by the user from informal supports, not the level of help *needed*. Section 2 of the CAN–M (R) is scored according to a sliding scale of help received, with the addition of a 'not known' option.

| | |
|---|---|
| **0 = None** | No help received from informal supports for this area of need |
| **1 = Low help** | The respondent perceives any support in this areas as being a little helpful |
| **2 = Moderate help** | The respondent perceives any support in this areas as being moderately helpful |
| **3 = High help** | The respondent perceives any support in this areas as being very helpful |
| **9 = Not known** | The respondent is unable to say how helpful informal supports have been in meeting needs |

## Section 3

Section 3 is completed only if a need (met or unmet) has been previously identified in Section 1. This section assesses the level of help provided by local services such as mental health workers, general practitioners, health visitors or social workers. In particular, the respondent is asked to indicate how helpful the local services have been in the past month in meeting her personal needs. For example, if the service user has received details of domestic violence programmes in the past month (low help), but states that this help has done nothing to meet her needs, then the perceived level of help needs to be rated as none (0). It is important to note that unlike Section 2, this section assesses both *received* help (Section 3*a*) and help that is needed by local services (Section 3*b*). This section has the same rating options as Section 2.

| | |
|---|---|
| **0 = None** | No help received from local services for this area of need |
| **1 = Low help** | The respondent perceives any support in this areas as being a little helpful |
| **2 = Moderate help** | The respondent perceives any support in this areas as being moderately helpful |
| **3 = High help** | The respondent perceives any support in this areas as being very helpful |
| **9 = Not known** | The respondent is unable to say how helpful local services have been in meeting needs |

## Section 4

This section is comprised of two separate questions. Section 4*a* assesses the respondent's perception of the appropriateness of interventions given by local services – that is, does she think that different help should be given? Section 4*b* examines whether the service user is satisfied with the amount of help she is receiving for meeting her needs – does she think that more help should be given? Both the service user and the keyworker are encouraged to provide an answer for Section 4*a*, whereas only the service user is invited to give a response to Section 4*b*. Staff are not asked to give an opinion to Section 4*b* as it could involve asking them to criticise their own work performance or the services that employ them. There are three rating options for each subsection:

| | |
|---|---|
| **0 = No** | **Section 4*a***: The respondent (service user or staff) believes the service user is not receiving the right type of help |
| | **Section 4*b***: The service user is not satisfied with the amount of help she is receiving |
| **1 = Yes** | **Section 4*a*:** The respondent (service user or staff) believes the service user is receiving the right type of help |
| | **Section 4*b***: The service user is satisfied with the amount of help she is receiving |
| **9 = Not known** | **Section 4*a*:** The respondent (service user or staff) is not able to say whether the service user is receiving the right type of help |
| | **Section 4*b***: The service user is not able to say whether she is satisfied with the amount of help she is receiving |

## Scoring the CAN–M (S)

The CAN–M (S) can be used for both clinical and research purposes and is found in Appendix 4. This version is a 1-page summary of the needs of pregnant women and mothers with SMI. It identifies 26 needs (met and unmet), as described in the previous chapter. The CAN–M (S) uses an identical rating system to that adopted in Section 1 of the CAN–M (C) and CAN–M (R), and therefore has five possible scoring options available (no need, met need, unmet need, not applicable and not known). Although suggested opening trigger questions for the service user interview are provided in italics, any of the prompt questions found in the CAN–M (C) may also be suitable for use with the CAN–M (S).

How CAN–M (S) information is used will depend on why the assessment is being made. Information can be used for at least three purposes:

(a)     CAN–M (S) data can be used at the level of the individual service user, by providing a baseline measure of level of need, or for charting changes over time.

(b)     CAN–M (S) data can be used for auditing and developing an individual service as described above under CAN–M (C).

(c)     CAN–M (S) data can be used as an outcome measure for research purposes such as the impact on needs of two different types of mental health services or the reasons why staff and service user perceptions differ.

# 8 Training for use of the CAN–M

## *Katherine Hunt and Louise Howard*

The CAN–M (C), CAN–M (R) and CAN–M (S) can be used by researchers and clinical staff. This chapter provides staff with training, including introducing the concept of needs assessment and providing practical exercises in the use of the CAN–M instrument. Suggested material for 12 overhead transparencies (Appendix 7) are provided below, along with issues to consider with each overhead.

Although extensive formal training is not necessary when using the CAN–M, an initial session such as the one presented below can be very useful in achieving several aims. It may help staff to understand the benefits of using a standardised instrument to assess needs, highlight that service users and staff often have different perceptions of need, and it may help staff to recognise that there are special issues that need consideration when working with pregnant women and mothers with SMI. Training sessions may also help to increase interrater reliability if being used for research purposes.

This chapter provides an outline of a 1–1½-hour informal training session with staff interaction. The length of the training session can be adjusted depending on the needs of each group. As the principles underlying rating for the CAN–M (C), CAN–M (R) and CAN–M (S) are the same, the training can focus on any of these versions. For CAN–M (C) and CAN–M (R) training, the rating sheets provided in Appendices 5 and 6 are used to record ratings of the four sections. For CAN–M (S) training, assessment summary score sheets are not required as the instrument is a self-contained document (Appendix 4). Training vignettes can be found in Appendix 8.

## Overhead transparencies

### 1. The Camberwell Assessment of Need for Mothers (CAN–M): aims of the session

- What are needs?
- Why assess needs?
- Benefits of using the CAN–M
- CAN–M administration and scoring
- Important issues to consider

---

**Discussion points (5 minutes)**

A general introduction to the CAN–M instrument is required here, in addition to information about the trainer's role, aims of the training session, and any expectations that the group may have of the session.

---

## 2. Needs assessment in pregnant women and mothers with severe mental illness

- Definition of need and importance of needs assessment

  'The requirements of individuals to enable them to achieve, maintain and restore an acceptable level of social independence or quality of life' (National Health Service and Community Care Act 1990)

- Services should be provided on the basis of need
- Everyone has needs arising from a variety of causes
- Need as a subjective concept
- Pregnant women and mothers with SMI have specific needs that may not be met by current services

---

**Discussion points (10 minutes)**

Concept of population-based and individual-based needs; provide a definition of need, such as the National Health Service and Community Care Act 1990, and ask the staff to brainstorm and share with the group examples of need.

Explain that services should be provided on the basis of need and that a need does not exist if there is no realistic intervention available.

Need is a subjective concept and therefore people may have differing but equally valid views as to whether a need exists or not.

There is a growing recognition that pregnant women and mothers with SMI have specific needs that may not be met by current services. A possible reason for this may relate to the absence to date of standardised assessment tools that systematically measure their needs.

---

## 3. Benefits of using the CAN–M

- Brief and user-friendly
- Comprehensive (26 domains)
- Incorporates both service user and staff views
- Records met and unmet needs
- Measures the help provided by informal supports and services separately
- Valid and reliable
- No formal training
- Suitable for research and clinical use

---

**Discussion points (10 minutes)**

This overhead serves to highlight that there are many benefits to revising the original CAN instrument with other populations. The CAN has been successfully revised with other populations, including the forensic population (CANFOR), people with learning and developmental disabilities (CANDID) and the elderly population (CANE).

The instruments belonging to the CAN family are brief and user-friendly. They take approximately 15–25 minutes to complete and avoid the use of medical jargon.

The CAN–M is a comprehensive assessment, covering many areas of need that are often neglected in other needs assessment tools. It recognises that both service users and staff views may vary, yet are equally valid. These different viewpoints are accommodated in the assessment in separate columns and should not be combined when completing the scales. These differences of opinion need to be considered when developing a care plan and may have an impact on the service user's commitment to treatment.

> **(Continued)**
> Met and unmet needs are recorded and the CAN–M (R) measures the level of help given and needed by both informal and formal services.
> The instrument has good interrater reliability, test–retest reliability, content validity and concurrent validity.
> The instrument can also be used in various research and clinical contexts.

## 4. CAN–M: need domains

1. Accommodation
2. Food
3. Looking after the home
4. Self-care
5. Daytime activities
6. General physical health
7. Pregnancy care
8. Sleep
9. Psychotic symptoms
10. Psychological distress
11. Information
12. Safety to self
13. Safety to child/children and others
14. Substance misuse
15. Company
16. Intimate relationships
17. Sexual health
18. Violence and abuse
19. Practical demands of childcare
20. Emotional demands of childcare
21. Basic education
22. Telephone
23. Transport
24. Budget
25. Benefits
26. Language, culture and religion

> **Discussion points (5 minutes)**
> This overhead provides a list of the 26 CAN–M domains. The domains cover a range of health, social and psychological needs that are relevant to pregnant women and mothers with SMI.
> Every domain is assessed in the same way, although three domains – *Pregnancy care*, *Practical demands of childcare* and *Emotional demands of childcare* – have the option of being rated as 'Not applicable'.

## 5. Introducing the CAN–M coversheet

- Information is collected about the service user, her children and the care coordinator
- The impact of the mother's mental state on the child must be considered *at all times*
- There is a need to break confidentiality if a child is thought to be at risk of harm
- Care coordinators and social workers are suitable professionals to contact if child protection issues are identified

> **Discussion points (10 minutes)**
> It is important that staff have an opportunity to familiarise themselves with the coversheet, which must be completed at the start of every interview.
> Highlight the importance of considering the mother's mental state on the child at all times, especially when unmet need, or moderate or high help, has been identified in the domains of *Self-care* (4), *Psychotic symptoms* (9), *Psychological distress* (10), *Safety to self* (12), *Safety to child/children and others* (13), *Substance misuse* (14), *Violence and abuse* (18), *Practical demands of childcare* (19), and the *Emotional demands of childcare* (20).

---

**(Continued)**

Invite the group to discuss when they think it would be appropriate to break confidentiality and how they would go about informing the mother of the need to disclose.

---

## 6. Introducing the four CAN–M sections: met and unmet needs

### Section 1

- Acts as a filter to determine the need for further assessment and provides an overall needs rating for the domain
    - i.   A need is met if the person has no problem or a mild to moderate problem in the domain, owing to the help given (rating 1)
    - ii.  A need is unmet if the person has a current serious problem in the domain, irrespective of help given (rating 2)
    - iii. There is no need if the person has no problem in the domain and no help is given (rating 0)
    - iv.  The rating is not known if the person does not know or does not wish to answer (rating 9)
    - v.   The question is not applicable to the service user (rating 8)

---

**Discussion points (10 minutes)**

This overhead introduces staff to the rating system used for identifying met and unmet needs with the CAN–M. This section is included in the CAN–M (R), the CAN–M (C)) and CAN–M (S) forms.

Emphasise the point that a need remains unmet if the person continues to have a serious problem, irrespective of the type and amount of help given.

Hand out a selection of CAN–M domains to the staff and draw their attention to the importance of using the anchor points in Section 1 to guide their answers.

The *Pregnancy care* domain is to be rated as 'Not applicable' if the mother has not recently given birth (within the past 12 months). The *Practical demands of childcare* and *Emotional demands of childcare* domains should also be rated as 'Not applicable' if the mother has no contact with her child.

---

## 7. Introducing the four CAN–M sections: help and satisfaction

### Section 2

- Assesses how much informal help from partner, friends and relatives has been received during the past month.

Rating key is identical for Sections 2 and 3.

    0 = no help
    1 = low help
    2 = moderate help
    3 = high help
    9 = not known

## Section 3

- Assesses current and required levels of support from services. It rates perceived levels of help received and the interviewee's perception of what help she actually needs

## Section 4

CAN–M (C)

- Records any other information
- Records action plan

CAN–M (R)

- Assesses the service user's overall satisfaction with the help she is currently receiving

Rating key:

0 = not satisfied
1 = satisfied
9 = not known

> **Discussion points (10 minutes)**
> Sections 2, 3 and 4 are in the CAN–M (R) and CAN–M (C) forms only, not the CAN–M (S).
> Section 2 assesses the level of help received by the service user from her partner, friends and relatives.
> Section 3 refers to any help currently received from local services, in addition to what help is needed from the local services for this area of need.
> Section 4 in CAN–M (R) asks the service user whether she believes she is receiving the right type of help for her needs and whether she is satisfied with the amount of help given. Staff are only asked whether they believe the user is receiving the right type of help for her needs. Section 4 in CAN–M (C) is a space for staff to record any other relevant

## *8. Other issues to consider when assessing the needs of pregnant women and mothers with severe mental illness*

- Motherhood is often an integral part of identity
- Fear of custody loss
- History of abuse
- Support of partner and extended family
- Involvement of specialist services, for example social services, perinatal services
- Stigma

> **Discussion points (10 minutes)**
> Pregnant women and mothers with SMI frequently encounter problems or experiences that require specific attention and sensitivity.
> Motherhood is often thought to be an integral part of women's identity, yet it is frequently overlooked and unrecognised by mental health services.
> Many of these women live in fear that their children may be removed from their care and therefore may be reluctant to disclose parenting difficulties.

**(Continued)**

A significant number of these women may have experienced violence and abuse either in childhood or as an adult. Abuse may include verbal threats, physical abuse, rape, and financial exploitation.

Partners and extended family may be viewed as valuable sources of support or as a major stressor or burden. It is important to explore with the mother what types of support she has available to her and whether they have a positive or negative influence on her life. Many of these women may have a number of professionals working to address their needs, but a lack of communication between professionals is often cited as a common source of stress for them.

Stigmatisation and the impact that it may have on their children is a constant worry for some of these mothers.

## 9. Scoring

- Summary score sheets
    - (a) Met needs (count the number of 1s)
    - (b) Unmet needs (count the number of 2s)
    - (c) Total needs (add number of met and unmet needs)

**Discussion points (5 minutes)**

Hand out copies of the CAN–M (R) or CAN–M (C) assessment summary sheet to allow staff the opportunity to familiarise themselves with the scoring form.

'Not applicable' (8) and 'Not known' (9) responses are to be rated as 'No needs' (0).

## 10. Case vignettes – rating needs using CAN–M (S)

- Read the vignettes
- Identify the needs according to the service user and staff
- Discuss whether the domains included are
    - (a) No need
    - (b) Met need
    - (c) Unmet need
    - (d) Not applicable
    - (e) Not known
- Where do staff and user views differ and how would you address the discrepancies?

**Discussion points (15–45 minutes)**

The purpose of the last two overhead transparicies is to provide staff with some practical experience using the CAN–M. It is recommended that the trainer go through the first CAN–M (S) vignette with the group, allowing them the opportunity to observe his/her decision-making process for identifying met and unmet needs. When the first vignette is completed, split the group into pairs and ask staff to enact role-plays using the remaining CAN–M (S) case vignettes, taking it in turns to be the interviewer and respondent.

Learning can be maximised by one pair enacting a role-play in front of the rest of the group and other staff then commenting on questioning style and scores.

Encourage the group to discuss how they would address any discrepancies between the service users and staff members' perceptions of met and unmet needs

## 11. Case vignettes – rating levels of help using CAN–M (R)

- Read the vignettes for the domains of *Pregnancy care*, *Safety to child/children and others*, and *Emotional demands of childcare*
- Identify the levels of support from formal and informal care, and whether the help provided is the right type and amount
- Where do staff and user views differ and how would you address the discrepancies?

---

**Discussion points (15 minutes)**

The final task is to provide the staff with some practical experience using Sections 2, 3 and 4 of the CAN–M (R) form.

Three important domains have been selected for this task; (1) *Pregnancy care*, (2) *Safety to child/children and others* and (3) *Emotional demands of childcare*.

Staff should be encouraged to fill out the CAN–M (R) assessment summary sheet and to share their answers with the rest of the group. Again, the group may like to discuss how they would address any discrepancies between the service users' and staff member's perception of met and unmet needs.

---

# Frequently asked questions

## What is the CAN–M?

The Camberwell Assessment of Need for Mothers, or CAN–M, is a revised version of the Camberwell Assessment of Needs (CAN). The instrument is designed to assess 26 health and social care problems experienced by pregnant women or mothers with SMI. It has been designed to identify rather than describe in detail the perceptions of both the service user and a member of staff. The CAN–M comes in three versions: a full clinical version, CAN–M (C); a full research version, CAN–M (R); and a short appraisal schedule, CAN–M (S).

## Who can use the CAN–M?

### Service users

Service users can be assessed using the CAN–M if they are of working age (18–65 years), pregnant and/ or have given birth to a child who is 16 years or younger.

### Professionals

Any person with experience of working with pregnant women and mothers with SMI, including nurses, social workers, psychologists, occupational therapists, psychiatrists, mental health workers, midwifes, obstetricians and health visitors, can use the CAN–M.

## Is the CAN–M accurate?

The CAN–M is a standardised instrument which has excellent interrater reliability (the extent to which two or more coders or interviewers agree), test–retest reliability (consistency over time), content validity (the extent to which we have sample-population representativeness) and concurrent validity (the accuracy of a measure or procedure by comparing it with another measure or procedure that has been demonstrated to be valid).

## What is the difference between a met and an unmet need?

A met need indicates that problems or difficulties have been identified for which effective help (either informal or formal) has been received in the past month. An unmet need indicates that problems or difficulties have been identified, irrespective of whether the person is receiving help for that problem.

## Is there any difference between scoring an item not applicable (a score of 8) and no problem (a score of 0)?

A 'not applicable' (8) response is available for three of the 26 CAN–M domains. When scoring the number of met needs, unmet needs and total needs, the score of 8 should be re-coded as 0, so as to maintain consistency with scoring of the other CAN instruments and to enable comparable results.

## If the person refuses to answer or it is obvious that their assessment is not accurate, can I correct the answer to reflect what is already known?

No. The ratings in each column must reflect the views of the respondents alone.

## How do I rate Section 3 if a service has been offered but the service user has refused it?

Section 3a assess the level of help received from local services. Service users who have been offered a particular service but have refused the intervention should be scored as 0, as no help has actually been received from their local services. Whether there is a need for this particular intervention, however, and whether the service user is receiving the right type of help can be documented in Sections 3b and 4.

## What if the service user refuses to answer a particular question?

Service users who refuse to answer questions should have their needs rated as not known (9). It is important not to push the service user into answering every question, especially if she does not feel comfortable with the sensitive nature of some of the questions.

## What if problems are identified in a particular domain for which there is no suitable intervention available locally?

Local availability of appropriate interventions is not used to determine the existence of a particular need. If a need exists for which there are no appropriate service interventions available, the domain should be recorded as 2 (an unmet need). Pregnant women and mothers with SMI often present with complex needs and the key worker must consider not only the needs of the mother but also the needs of the child at all times. Unmet needs in particular domains may indicate a failure of multi-agency collaboration, such as social services working in partnership with adult mental health services, or the need to recruit workers with expertise in particular areas of assessment and intervention.

### When is the 'Pregnancy care' domain applicable?

When a service user has confirmatory evidence that she is pregnant. Generally speaking, this domain is applicable until about 12 months post-partum. However, if the respondent states there are ongoing physical complications as a result of her pregnancy or birth, then rate the service user as having needs irrespective of the time since birth.

### What if the mother does not have any contact with the child? Is the CAN–M still an appropriate instrument?

Yes. The CAN–M is a suitable instrument for service users who have either full custody of their child, limited visiting rights, or who have no contact with the child. In the last case, however, domain 19 (*Practical demands of childcare*) and domain 20 (*Emotional demands of childcare*) should be considered as not applicable (8).

### What should I do if I have concerns about child protection issues?

If there are child protection concerns, these should be discussed with a supervisor or manager. If, after this discussion, there are concerns that the child is at suspected or identified risk, this should be discussed with the mother's care coordinator and/or social services.

### What should I do if the service user discloses acts of violence and abuse against her?

It is important to establish the safety of service users. If the service user reports current domestic violence then it will be important to ensure that she has all the necessary information to allow her to take a decision about whether to stay with or to leave her partner. At the very least, the contact details of local safe houses and women's support agencies should be given. If a child is being exposed to these acts of violence and abuse, however, either directly or indirectly in the home, this should be viewed as a child protection issue and discussed with a manager.

### Can I add additional need domains to the CAN–M such as body image?

Yes, other need domains can be added, but the reliability and validity of these extra domains have not been established. Also, they should not be used as a substitute for existing domains or included in the recommended scoring methods.

### Can I translate CAN–M into another language for use in my service?

The authors would encourage this collaboration and would like to hear from colleagues interested in discussing possible translations. They can be contacted at the address below.

## Do you need any formal training in order to be able to use the CAN–M?

Although previous clinical training is not necessary for the CAN–M, people should be familiar with the administration and scoring procedures before using it. People should also be familiar with some of the more common problems faced by pregnant women and mothers with SMI, as well as having a good understanding of what action needs to be taken if a woman discloses that either herself or others (in particular children) are at risk of harm.


## What do I do if my question has not been answered?

Write your question to:

> CAN–M,
> Section of Community Mental Health,
> Health Service and Population Research Department,
> Institute of Psychiatry,
> Denmark Hill,
> London SE5 8AF
> UK

# References

Ackerson, B. J. (2003) Coping with the dual demands of severe mental illness and parenting: the parent's perspective. *Families in Society: The Journal of Contemporary Human Services*, **84**, 109–118.

Ainsworth, M., Blehar, M., Waters, E., *et al* (1978) *Patterns of Attachment: A Psychological Study of the Strange Situation*. Lawrence Erlbaum

Alder, J., Fink, N., Bitzer, J., *et al* (2007). Depression and anxiety during pregnancy: a risk factor for obstetric, foetal and neonatal outcome? A critical review of the literature. *The Journal of Maternal Foetal and Neonatal Medicine*, **20**, 189–209.

Aldridge, J. & Becker, S. (2003) *Children Caring for Parents with Mental Illness: Perspectives of Young Carers, Parents and Professionals*. The Policy Press.

Amaro, H., Fried, L. E., Cabral, H., *et al* (1990) Violence during pregnancy and substance use. *American Journal of Public Health*, **80**, 575–579.

Anderson, C. M., Hogarty, G. E. & Reiss, D. J. (1980) Family treatment of adult schizophrenic patients: a psychoeducational approach. *Schizophrenia Bulletin*, **6**, 490–505.

Andresen, R., Caputi, P. & Oades, L. G. (2000) Interrater reliability of the Camberwell Assessment of Need Short Appraisal Schedule. *Australian and New Zealand Journal of Psychiatry*, **34**, 856–861.

Anthony, E. J. (1976) How children cope in families with a psychotic parent. In *Infant Psychiatry: A New Synthesis* (eds E. N. Rexford, L. W. Sander & T. Shapiro). Yale University Press.

Apfel, R. J. & Handel, M. H. (1993) *Madness and Loss of Motherhood: Sexuality, Reproduction and Long-term Mental Illness*. American Psychiatric Press.

Arvidsson, H. (2001) Needs assessed by patients and staff in a Swedish sample of severely mentally ill subjects. *Nordic Journal of Psychiatry*, **55**, 311–317.

Arvidsson, H. (2003) Test–retest reliability of the Camberwell Assessment of Need (CAN). *Nordic Journal of Psychiatry*, **57**, 279–283.

Ashaye, O. A., Livingston, G. & Orrell, M. W. (2003) Does standardized needs assessment improve the outcome of psychiatric day hospital care for older people? A randomized controlled trial. *Aging and Mental Health*, **7**, 195–199.

Bacchus, L., Mezey, G. & Bewley, S. (2003) Experiences of seeking help from health professionals in a sample of women who experienced domestic violence. *Health and Social Care in the Community*, **11**, 10–18.

Barnardo's (2004) *Keeping The Family In Mind. A Briefing on Young Carers Whose Parents Have Mental Health Problems*. (http://barnardos.org.uk/keeping_the_family_in_mind.pdf).

Bassett, H., Lampe, J. & Lloyd, C. (1999) Parenting: experiences and feelings of parents with mental illness. *Journal of Mental Health*, **8**, 597–604.

Bassuk, E. L., Weinreb, L. F., Buckner, J. C., *et al* (1996) The characteristics and needs of sheltered homeless and low income housed mothers. *JAMA*, **276**, 640–646.

Bassuk, E. L., Buckner, J. C., Perloff, J. N., *et al* (1998) Prevalence of mental health and substance use disorders among homeless and low income housed mothers. *American Journal of Psychiatry*, **155**, 1561–1564.

Beardslee, W. R., Versage, E. M., Gladstone, T. R. (1998) Children of affectively ill parents: a review of the past 10 years. *Journal of the American Academy of Child and Adolescent Psychiatry*, **37**, 1134–1141.

Bebbington, P. (1992) Assessing the need for psychiatric treatment at the district level: the need for surveys. In *Measuring Mental Health Needs* (eds G. Thornicroft, C. Brewin & J. Wing), pp. 99–117. Royal College of Psychiatrists.

Beidel, D. C. & Turner, S. M. (1997) At risk for anxiety: 1 Psychopathology in the offspring of anxious parents. *Journal of the American Academy of Child and Adolescent Psychiatry*, **36**, 918–924.

Belle, D. (ed.) (1982) *Lives in Stress: Women and Depression*. Sage Publications.

Bennedsen, R. E., Mortensen, P. B. & Olesen, A. V. (1999) Preterm birth and intra-uterine growth retardation among children of women with schizophrenia. *British Journal of Psychiatry*, **175**, 239–245.

Bennedsen, B. E., Mortensen, P. B. & Olesen, A. V., *et al* (2001) Congenital malformations, stillbirths, and infant deaths among children of women with schizophrenia. *Archives of General Psychiatry*, **58**, 674–679.

Black, C., Bucky, S. F. & Wilder-Padilla, S. (1986) The interpersonal and emotional consequences of being an adult child of an alcoholic. *The International Journal of the Addictions*, **21**, 213–321.

Black, R. & Mayer, J. (1980) Parents with special problems: alcoholism and opiate addiction. *Child Abuse and Neglect*, **4**, 45–54.

Blanch, A. K., Nicholson, J. & Purcell, J. (1994) Parents with severe mental illness and their children: the need for human services integration. *The Journal of Health Administration*, **21**, 388–396.

Bonari, L., Pinto, N., Ahn, E., *et al* (2004) Perinatal risks of untreated depression during pregnancy. *Canadian Journal of Psychiatry*, **49**, 726–735.

Bornstein, M. H., Bradley, R. H. & von Eye, A. (eds) (2003) *Socioeconomic Status, Parenting and Child Development*. Lawrence Erlbaum Associates.

Bowen, E., Heron, J., Waylen, A., *et al* (2005) Domestic violence risk during and after pregnancy: findings from a British longitudinal study. *British Journal of Gynaecology*, **112**, 1083–1089.

Bradshaw, J. (1972) A taxonomy of social need. In *Problems and Progress in Medical Care: Essays on Current Research* (J. McLachlan ed.), pp. 69–82. Oxford University Press.

Brewin, C., Wing, J., Mangen, S., *et al* (1987) Principles and practice of measuring needs in the long-term mentally ill: the MRC Needs for Care Assessment. *Psychological Medicine*, **17**, 971–981.

Brewin, C., Wing, J. & Mangen, S. (1988) Needs for care among the long-term mentally ill: a report from the Camberwell High Contact Survey. *Psychological Medicine*, **18**, 457–468.

Brown, G. W. & Harris, T. (1978) *Social Origins of Depression: A Study of Psychiatric Disorders in Women*. Tavistock.

Browne, K. & Herbert, M. (1997) *Preventing Family Violence*. John Wiley & Sons.

Buist, A. E., Dennerstein, L. & Burrows, G. D. (1990) Review of a mother–baby unit in a psychiatric hospital. *Australian and New Zealand Journal of Psychiatry*, **24**, 103–108.

Bybee, D., Mowbray, C. T., Oyserman, D., *et al* (2003) Variability in community functioning of mothers with severe mental illness. *Journal of Behavioural Health Services Research*, **30**, 269–289.

Cadoret, R. J., Yates, W. R., Troughton, E., *et al* (1995) Genetic–environmental interaction in the genesis of aggressivity and conduct disorders. *Archives of General Psychiatry*, **52**, 916–924.

Carlson, G. A. & Weintraub, S. (1993) Childhood behaviour problems and bipolar disorder: relationship or coincidence? *Journal of Affective Disorders*, **28**, 143–153.

Carter, M., Crosby, C., Geerthuis, S., *et al* (1996) Developing reliability in client-centred mental health needs assessment. *Journal of Mental Health*, **5**, 233–243.

Cascardi, M., Mueser, K. T., De Giralomo J., *et al* (1996) Physical aggression against psychiatric inpatients by family members and partners. *Psychiatric Services*, **47**, 531–533.

Caton, C. L., Cournos, F., Felix, A., *et al* (1998) Childhood experiences and current adjustment of offspring of indigent patients with schizophrenia. *Psychiatric Services*, **49**, 86–90.

Clark, K. A., Martin, S. L., Peterson, R., *et al* (2000) Who gets screened during pregnancy for partner violence? *Archives of Family Medicine*, **9**, 1093–1099.

Cogan, J. C. (1998) The consumer as expert: women with serious mental illness and their relationship-based needs. *Psychiatric Rehabilitation Journal*, **22**, 142–154.

Cogan, N., Riddell, S. & Mayes, G. (2004) Children living with mental health problems. In *Thriving, Surviving or Going Under: Coping with Everyday Lives Series, Research on Stress and Coping in Education* (E. Frydenberg ed.). Information Age Publishing.

Coghill, S. R., Caplan, H. L., Alexandra, H., *et al* (1986) Impact of post-natal depression on cognitive development in young children. *BMJ*, **292**, 1165–1167.

Cohen, L. S. & Rosenbaum, J.F. (1998) Psychotropic drug use during pregnancy: weighing the risks. *Journal of Clinical Psychiatry*, **59** (Suppl 2), 18–28.

Cohen, L. S., Altshuler, L. L., Harlow, B. L., *et al* (2006) Relapse of major depression during pregnancy in women who maintain or discontinue antidepressant medication. *JAMA*, **295**, 499–507.

Confidential Enquiry into Maternal and Child Health (CEMACH) (2004) Why Mothers Die 2000–2002. The Sixth Confidential Enquiry into Maternal Deaths. CEMACH.

Cooper, P. J. & Murray, L. (1998) Postnatal depression. *BMJ*, **316**, 1884–1886.

Coverdale, J. H. & Aruffo, J. A. (1989) Family planning needs of female chronic psychiatric patients. *American Journal of Psychiatry*, **146**, 1489–1491.

Cox, A. D., Puckering, C., Pound, A., *et al* (1987) The impact of maternal depression in young children. *Child Psychology and Psychiatry*, **28**, 917–928.

Cox, A. D., Puckering, C., Pound, A., *et al* (1991) Evaluation of a lone visiting befriending service for young mothers: NEWPIN. *Journal of the Royal College of Medicine*, **84**, 217–220.

Dawson, G., Frey, K., Panagiotides, H., *et al* (1997) Infants of depressed mothers exhibit atypical frontal brain activity: A replication and extension of previous findings. *Journal of Child Psychology and Psychiatry*, **38**, 179–186.

Dearden, C. & Becker, S. (2000) *Growing Up Caring: Vulnerability and Transition to Adulthood – Young Carers' Experiences*. Youth Work Press.

DeChillo, N., Matorin, S. & Hallahan, C. (1987) Children of psychiatric patients: rarely seen or heard. *Health and Social Work*, **12**, 296–302.

Department of Health (1990) *National Health Service and Community Care Act*. TSO (The Stationary Office).

Department of Health (1995) *Mental Health in England:1982–1992*. Government Statistical Service..

Department of Health (1999a) *Mental Health Act 1983. Code of Practice*. TSO (The Stationary Office)

Department of Health (1999b) *Mental Health National Service Framework*. TSO (The Stationary Office).

Department of Health (2002) *Women's Mental Health: Into the Mainstream. Strategic Development of Mental Health Care for Women*. (http://www.dh.gov.uk/en/Consultations/Closedconsultations/DH_4075478). Department of Health.

Department of Health (2003) *Mainstreaming Gender and Women's Mental Health: Implementation Guidance*. (http://www.dh.gov.uk/en/Publicationsandstatistics/Publications/PublicationsPolicyAndGuidance/DH_4072067). Department of Health.

Department of Health (2006) *Responding to Domestic Abuse: A Handbook for Health Professionals*. (http://www.dh.gov.uk/prod_consum_dh/groups/dh_digitalassets/@dh/@en/documents/digitalasset/dh_4126619.pdf). Department of Health.

Diav-Citrin, O., Schechtman, S., Ornoy, S., *et al* (2005). Safety of haloperidol and penfluridol in pregnancy: a multicentre, prospective, controlled study. *Journal of Clinical Psychiatry*, **66**, 317–322.

Diaz-Caneja, A. & Johnson, S. (2004) The views and experiences of severely mentally ill mothers – a qualitative study. *Social Psychiatry and Psychiatric Epidemiology*, **39**, 472–482.

Dienemann, J., Boyle, E., Baker, D., *et al* (2000) Intimate partner abuse among women diagnosed with depression. *Issues in Mental Health Nursing*, **21**, 499–513.

Dipple, H., Smith, S., Andrews, H., *et al* (2002) The experience of motherhood in women with severe and enduring mental illness. *Journal of Social Psychiatry and Psychiatric Epidemiology*, **37**, 336–340.

d'Orban, P. T. (1979) Women who kill their children. *British Journal of Psychiatry*, **134**, 560–571.

Egami, Y., Ford, D. E., Greenfield, S. F., *et al* (1996) Psychiatric profile and sociodemographic characteristics of adults who report physically abusing or neglecting children. *American Journal of Psychiatry*, **153**, 921–928.

El Kady, D., Gilbert, W. M., Xing, G., *et al* (2005) Maternal and neonatal outcomes of assaults during pregnancy. *Obstetric Gynaecology*, **105**, 357–363.

Emery, R., Weintraub, S. & Neale, J. M. (1982) Effects of marital discord on the school behaviour of children of schizophrenic, affectively disordered, and normal patients. *Journal of Abnormal Child Psychology*, **10**, 215–228.

Endicott, J., Spitzer, R. L., Fleiss, J. L., *et al* (1976) The Global Assessment Scale: a procedure for measuring overall severity of psychiatric disturbance. *Archives of General Psychiatry*, **33**, 766–771.

Ensminger, M. E., Hanson, S. G., Riley, A. W., *et al* (2003) Maternal psychological distress: adult sons' and daughters' mental health and educational attainment. *Journal of American Academic Child and Adolescent Psychiatry*, **42**, 1108–1115.

Evans, S., Greenhalgh, J. & Connelly, J. (2000) Selecting a mental health needs assessment scale: guidance on the critical appraisal of standardized measures. *Journal of Evaluation in Clinical Practice*, **6**, 379–393.

Falkov, A. (1996) *A Study of Working Together 'Part 8 Reports': Fatal Child Abuse and Parental Psychiatric Disorder*. Department of Health.

Falkov, A. (1997) *Parental Psychiatric Disorder and Child Maltreatment Part 2: Extent and Nature of the Association (Highlight Series No. 149)*. National Children's Bureau.

Falloon, I. R. (2000) Problem solving as a core strategy in the prevention of schizophrenia and other mental disorders. *Australian and New Zealand Journal of Psychiatry*, **34** (Suppl), 185–190.

Famularo, R., Kinscherff, R. & Fenton, T. (1992) Parental substance abuse and the nature of child maltreatment. *Child Abuse and Neglect*, **16**, 475–483.

Feldman, R., Weller, A., Leckman, J. F., *et al* (1999) The nature of the mother's tie to her infant: maternal bonding under conditions of proximity, separation and potential loss. *Journal of Reproductive and Infant Psychology*, **40**, 929–939.

Fitzgerald, H. E., Puttler, L. I., Mun, E. Y., *et al* (2000) Prenatal and postnatal exposure to parental alcohol use and abuse. In *WAIMH Handbook of Infant Mental Health Volume 4: Infant Mental Health in Groups at High Risk* (eds J.D. Osofsky and H.E. Fitzgerald). John Wiley & Sons.

Flynn, S., Shaw, J. J. & Abel, K. M. (2007) Homicide of infants: a cross-sectional study. *Journal of Clinical Psychiatry*, **68**, 1501–1509.

Focht-Birkerts, L. & Beardslee, W. R. (2000) A child's experience of parental depression: encouraging relational resilience in families with affective illness. *Family Process*, **39**, 417–434.

Foley, D. L., Pickles, A., Simonoff, E., *et al* (2001) Parental concordance and co-morbidity for psychiatric disorder and associated risks for current psychiatric symptoms and disorders in a community sample of juvenile twins. *Journal of Child Psychology and Psychiatry*, **42**, 381–394.

Forbes, E. E., Shaw, D. S., Fox, N. A., *et al* (2006) Maternal depression, child frontal asymmetry, and child affective behaviour as factors in child behaviour problems. *Journal of Child Psychology and Psychiatry*, **47**, 79–87.

Foy, R., Nelson, F., Penney, G., *et al* (2000) Antenatal detection of domestic violence. *Lancet*, **355**, 1915.

Freeman, M. P., Gracious, B. L. & Wisner, K. L. (2002) Pregnancy outcomes in schizophrenia. *American Journal of Psychiatry*, **159**, 609.

Gandhi, S. G., Gilbert, W. M., McElyy, S. S., *et al* (2006) Maternal and neonatal outcomes after attempted suicide. *Obstetric Gynaecology*, **107**, 984–990.

Gazmararian, J. A., Lazorick, S., Spitz, A. M., *et al* (1996) Prevalence of violence against pregnant women. *JAMA*, **275**, 1915–1920.

Ge, X., Conger, R. D., Cadoret, R. J., *et al* (1996) The developmental interface between nature and nurture: a mutual influence model of child antisocial behaviour and parent behaviours. *Developmental Psychology*, **32**, 574–589.

Gelles, R. J. (1973) Child abuse as psychopathology: a sociological critique and reformulation. *American Journal of Orthopsychiatry*, **43**, 611–621.

Goldman, H. H. (1982) Mental illness and family burden: a public health perspective. *Hospital Community Psychiatry*, **33**, 557–560.

Goodman, S. H. (1987) Emory University project on children of disturbed parents. *Schizophrenia Bulletin*, **13**, 411–423.

Goodman, S. H. & Emory, E. K. (1992) Perinatal complications in births to low socio-economic status schizophrenic and depressed women. *Journal of Abnormal Psychology*, **101**, 225–229.

Goodyer, I., Kolvin, I. & Gatzanis, S. (1985) Recent undesirable life events and psychiatric disorder in childhood and adolescence. *British Journal of Psychiatry*, **147**, 517–523.

Goodyer, I. M., Cooper, P. J., Vize, C. M., *et al* (1993) Depression in 11–16 year old girls: the role of past parental psychopathology and exposure to recent life events. *Journal of Child Psychology and Psychiatry*, **34**, 1103–1115.

Gopfert, M., Webster, J. & Seeman, M. V. (eds) (1996) *Parental Psychiatric Disorder: Distressed Parents and Their Children*. Cambridge University Press.

Greenfield, S. F., Swartz, M. S., Landerman, L. R., *et al* (1993) Long-term psychosocial effects of childhood exposure to parental problem drinking. *American Journal of Psychiatry*, **150**, 608–613.

Gunnar, M. R. (1998) Quality of early care and buffering of neuroendocrine stress reactions: potential effects on the developing brain. *Preventative Medicine*, **27**, 208–211.

Hansson, L., Vinding, H. R., Mackeprang, T., *et al* (2001) Comparison of key worker and patient assessment of needs in schizophrenic patients living in the community: a Nordic multicentre study. *Acta Psychiatrica Scandinavica*, **103**, 45–51.

Hansson, L., Sandlund, M., Bengtsson-Tops, A., *et al* (2003) The relationship of needs and quality of life in persons with schizophrenia living in the community. A Nordic multi-center study. *Nordic Journal of Psychiatry*, **57**, 5–11.

Hawton, K., Roberts, J. & Goodwin, G. (1985) The risk of child abuse among mothers who attempt suicide. *British Journal of Psychiatry*, **146**, 486–489.

Heron, J., Robertson Blackmore, E., McGuinness, M., *et al* (2007) No 'latent period' in the onset of bipolar affective puerperal psychosis. *Archives of Women's Mental Health*, **10**, 79–81.

Hogg, L. & Marshall, M. (1992) Can we measure need in the homeless mentally ill? Using the MRC Needs for Care Assessment in hostels for the homeless. *Psychological Medicine*, **22**, 1027–1034.

Hollingsworth, L. D. (2004) Child custody loss among women with persistent severe mental illness. *Social Work Research*, **28**, 199–209.

Howard, L. M. (2005) Fertility and pregnancy in women with psychotic disorders. *European Journal of Obstetrics and Gynecology and Reproductive Biology*, **119**, 3–10.

Howard, L. M., Kumar, R. & Thornicroft, G. (2001) Psychosocial characteristics and needs of mothers with psychotic disorders. *British Journal of Psychiatry*, **178**, 427–432.

Howard, L. M., Leese, M., Kumar, C., *et al* (2002) The general fertility rate in women with psychotic disorders. *American Journal of Psychiatry*, **159**, 991–997.

Howard, L. M., Goss, C., Leese, M., *et al* (2003a) The medical outcome of pregnancy in women with psychotic disorders and their infants after birth. *British Journal of Psychiatry*, **182**, 63–67.

Howard, L. M., Shah, N., Salmon, M., *et al* (2003b) Predictors of parenting difficulties in women admitted to mother and baby units. *Social Psychology and Psychiatric Epidemiology*, **38**, 450–455.

Howard, L. M., Leese, M., Goss, C., *et al* (2004) The psychosocial outcome of pregnancy in women with psychotic disorders and for their infants in the first year postpartum. *Schizophrenia Research*, **71**, 49–60.

Howard, L. M., Hunt, K., Slade, M., *et al* (2007) Assessing the needs of pregnant women and mothers with severe mental illness: the psychometric properties of the Camberwell Assessment of Need – Mothers (CAN–M). *International Journal of Methods in Psychiatric Research*, **16**, 177–185.

Hunter, R., McLean, J., Peck, D., *et al* (2004) The Scottish 700 Outcomes Study: a comparative evaluation of the Health of the Nation Outcome Scale (HoNOS), the Avon Mental Health Measure (AVON), and an idiographic scale (OPUS) in adult mental health. *Journal of Mental Health*, **13**, 93–105.

Jablensky, A. V., Morgan, V., Zubrick, S. R., *et al* (2005) Pregnancy, delivery, and neonatal complications in a population cohort of women with schizophrenia and major affective disorders. *American Journal of Psychiatry*, **162**, 79–91.

Jaenicke, C., Hammen, C., Zupan, B., *et al* (1987) Cognitive vulnerability in children at risk for depression. *Journal of Abnormal Psychology*, **15**, 559–572.

Jarmas, A. L. & Kazak, A. E. (1992) Young adult children of alcoholic fathers: depressive experiences, coping styles and family systems. *Journal of Consulting and Clinical Psychology*, **60**, 244–251.

Johnson, J. G., Cohen, P., Kasen, S., *et al* (2001) Association of maladaptive parental behaviour with psychiatric disorder among parents and their offspring. *Archives of General Psychiatry*, **58**, 453–460.

Jones, I. & Craddock, N. (2001) Familiality of the puerperal trigger in bipolar disorder: results of a family study. *American Journal of Psychiatry*, **158**, 913–917.

Joseph, J. G., Joshi, S. V., Lewin, A., *et al* (1999) Characteristics and perceived needs of mothers with serious mental illness. *Psychiatric Services*, **50**, 1357–1359.

Junghan, U., Leese, M., Priebe, S., *et al* (2007) Staff and patient perspectives on unmet need and therapeutic alliance in community services. *British Journal of Psychiatry*, **191**, 543–    547.

Kaufman, C., Grunebaum, H., Cohler, B., *et al* (1979) Superkids: competent children of psychotic mothers. *American Journal of Psychiatry*, **136**, 1398–1402.

Kelly, R. H., Danielsen, B. H., Zatrick, D. F., *et al* (1999) Chart-recorded psychiatric diagnoses in women giving birth in California in 1992. *American Journal of Psychiatry*, **156**, 955–957.

Kendler, K. S., Neale, M. S., Kessler, R. C., *et al* (1992) Major depression and generalised anxiety disorder. Same genes (partly) different environments? *Archives of General Psychiatry*, **49**, 716–722.

Klimes-Dougan, B., Free, K., Ronsaville, D., *et al* (1999) Suicidal ideation and attempts: a longitudinal investigation of children of depressed and well mothers. *Journal of the American Academy of Child and Adolescent Psychiatry*, **38**, 686–692.

Korkeila, J., Heikkila, J., Hansson, L., *et al* (2005) Structure of needs among people with schizophrenia. *Social Psychiatry and Psychiatric Epidemiology*, **44**, 233–239.

Kornegay, C. J., Vasilakis-Scaramozza, C. & Jick, H. (2002) Incident diabetes associated with antipsychotic use in the United Kingdom general practice research database. *Journal of Clinical Psychiatry*, **63**, 758–762.

Krumm, S. & Becker, T. (2006) Subjective views of motherhood in women with mental illness – a sociological perspective. *Journal of Mental Health*, **15**, 449–460.

Kuperman, S., Schlosser, S. S., Lidral, J., *et al* (1999) Relationship of child psychopathology to parental alcoholism and antisocial personality disorder. *Journal of the American Academy of Child and Adolescent Psychiatry*, **38**, 686–692.

Kurstjens, S. & Wolke, D. (2001) Effects of maternal depression on cognitive development of children over the first seven years of life. *Journal of Child Psychology and Psychiatry*, **42**, 623–636.

Langrock, A. M., Compas, B. E., Keller, G., *et al* (2002) Coping with the stress of parental depression: parents' reports of children's coping emotional and behavioural problems. *Journal of Clinical Child and Adolescent Psychology*, **31**, 312–324.

Lasalvia, A., Ruggeri ,M., Mazzi, M. A., *et al* (2000) The perception of needs for care in staff and patients in community-based mental health services. The South Verona Outcome Project 3. *Acta Psychiatrica Scandinavica*, **102**, 366–375.

Lee, C. M. & Gotlib, I. H. (1989) Clinical Status and Emotional adjustment in depressed mothers. *American Journal of Psychiatry*, **146**, 478–483.

Lelliott, P. (2000) What do people want from specialist mental health services and can this be routinely measured in routine service settings? *Behavioural and Cognitive Psychotherapy*, **28**, 361–368.

Lesage, A., Mignolli, G. & Faccincani, C. (1991) Standardised assessment of the needs for care in a cohort of patients with schizophrenic psychoses. *Psychological Medicine*, **19** (suppl), 426–431.

Lewis, G. (2007) *Saving Mothers' Lives: Reviewing maternal deaths to make motherhood safer –2003–2005. The Seventh Report of the Confidential Enquiries into Maternal Deaths in the United Kingdom*. Confidential Enquiry into Maternal and Child Health.

Lin, L. I. (1989) A concordance correlation coefficient to evaluate reproducibility. *Biometrics*, **45**, 255–268.

Lindenmayer, J. P., Czobor, P., Volavka, J., *et al* (2003) Changes in glucose and cholesterol levels in patients with schizophrenia treated with typical or atypical antipsychotics. *American Journal of Psychiatry*, **160**, 290–296.

Littleton, H. L., Breitkopf, C. R. & Berenson, A. B. (2007) Correlates of anxiety symptoms during pregnancy and association with perinatal outcomes: a meta-analysis. *American Journal of Obstetrics and Gynaecology*, **196**, 424–432.

Lockwood, A. & Marshall, M. (1999) Can a standardized needs assessment be used to improve the care of people with severe mental disorders? A pilot study of 'needs feedback'. *Journal of Advanced Nursing*, **30**, 1408–1415.

MacDonald, S., Halliday, J. & MacEwan, T. (2003) Nithsdale Schizophrenia Surveys 24: sexual dysfunction. Case–control study. *British Journal of Psychiatry*, **182**, 50–66.

Markovitz, P. (1996) *The Avon Mental Health Measure*. Changing Minds.

Marks, M. N. & Kumar, R. (1993) Infanticide in England and Wales. *Medicine Science and the Law*, **33**, 329–339.

Marshall, M., Hogg, L., Gath, D. H., *et al* (1995) The Cardinal Needs Schedule: a modified version of the MRC Needs for Care Schedule. *Psychological Medicine*, **25**, 605–617.

Marshall, M., Lockwood, A., Green, G., *et al* (2004) Systematic assessments of need and care planning in severe mental illness: Cluster randomised controlled trial. *British Journal of Psychiatry*, **185**, 163–168.

Martin, S. L., Kilgallen, B., Dee, D. L., *et al* (1998) Women in a prenatal care/substance abuse treatment program: links between domestic violence and mental health. *Maternal Child Health Journal*, **2**, 85–94.

Maslow, A. (1954) *Motivation and Personality*. Harper & Row.

Mathew, R. J., Wilson, W. H., Blazer, D. G., *et al* (1993) Psychiatric disorders in adult children of alcoholics: data from the epidemiological catchment area project. *American Journal of Psychiatry*, **150**, 793–800.

McCrone, P., Leese, M., Thornicroft, G., *et al* (2000) Reliability of the Camberwell Assessment of Need – European Version. EPSILON Study 6. *British Journal of Psychiatry*, **177**, s34–s40.

McGrath, J. J., Hearle, J., Jenner, L., *et al* (1999) The fertility and fecundity of patients with psychoses. *Acta Psychiatrica Scandinavica*, **99**, 441–446.

McLean, K. T., Minkovitz, C. S., Strobino, D. M., *et al* (2006) The timing of maternal depressive symptoms and mother's parenting practices with young children: implications for paediatric practice. *Pediatrics*, **118**, 174–182.

McLoyd, V. C. (1998) Socioeconomic disadvantage and child development. *The American Psychologist*, **53**, 185–204.

Meltzer, H., Gill, B., Pettigrew, M., *et al* (1995) *The Prevalence of Psychiatric Morbidity Among Adults Aged 16–64 Living in Private Households in Great Britain. OPCS Surveys. Report 1.* Department of Health.

Meltzer, H., Gatwood, R., Goodman, R., *et al* (2000) *The Mental Health of Children and Adolescents in Great Britain.* Office for National Statistics.

Mental Health Branch (1997) *National Mental Health Report 6 1996: 4th Annual Report. Changes in Australia's Mental Health Services Under the National Mental Health Strategy.* Commonwealth Department of Health and Family Services.

Miller, L.J. & Finnerty, M. (1996) Sexuality, pregnancy, and childbearing among women with schizophrenia-spectrum disorders. *Psychiatric Services*, **47**, 502–505.

Mind (1997) *Mental Health Statistics*. Mind.

Moss, K. (2003). Witnessing violence – aggression and anxiety in young children. *Health Report*, **14**, 53–66.

Mowbray, C. T., Oyserman, D., Zemencuk, J. K., *et al* (1995) Motherhood for women with serious mental illness. *American Journal of Orthopsychiatry*, **65**, 21–38.

Mowbray, C. T., Schwartz, S., Bybee, D., *et al* (2000) Mothers with a mental illness: stressors and resources for parenting and living. *Families in Society: Journal of Contemporary Human Services*, **81**, 118–129.

Mowbray, C. T., Oyserman, D., MacFarlane, P., *et al* (2001) Life circumstances of mothers with serious mental illness. *Psychiatric Rehabilitation Journal*, **25**, 114–123.

Mowbray, C. T., Bybee, D., Hollingsworth, L., *et al* (2005a) Living arrangements and social support: effects on the well-being of mothers with mental illness. *Social Work Research*, **29**, 41–55.

Mowbray, C. T., Bybee, D., Oyserman, D., *et al* (2005b) Timing of mental illness onset and motherhood. *Journal of Nervous Mental Disorders*, **193**, 369–378.

Mullick, M., Miller, L.J. & Jacobsen, T. (2001) Insight into mental illness and child maltreatment risk among mothers with major psychiatric disorders. *Psychiatric Services*, **52**, 488–492.

Munk-Olsen, T., Laursen, T. M., Pedersen, C. B., *et al* (2006) New parents and mental disorders: a population-based register stidy. *JAMA*, **296**, 2582–2589.

Murray, L., Sinclair, D., Cooper, P., *et al* (1999) The socio-emotional development of 5-year old children of postnatally depressed mothers. *Journal of Child Psychology and Psychiatry*, **40**, 1259–1271.

National Health Service and Community Care Act 1990. TSO (The Stationery Office).

National Institute for Health and Clinical Excellence (2007) *Antenatal and Postnatal Mental Health: Clinical Management and Service Guidance*. National Institute for Health and Clinical Excellence

Nicholson, J., Sweeney, E. M. & Geller, J. L. (1998a) Mothers with mental illness. The competing demands of parenting and living with mental illness. *Psychiatric Services*, **49**, 635–642.

Nicholson, J., Sweeney, E. M. & Geller, J. L. (1998b) Mothers with mental illness: Family relationships and the context of parenting. *Psychiatric Services*, **49**, 643–649.

O'Connor, T. G., Deater-Deckard, K., Fulker, D., *et al* (1998) Genotype–environment correlations in late childhood and early adolescence: antisocial behavioural problems and coercive parenting. *Developmental Psychology*, **34**, 970–981.

O'Keane, V., Marsh, M. & Seneriatne, G. (eds) (2006) Mood disorder during pregnancy. In *Psychiatric Disorders in Pregnancy: Obstetric and Psychiatric Care*. Martin Dunitz.

O'Leary, D. & Webb, M. (1996) The needs for care assessment – a longitudinal approach. *Psychiatric Bulletin*, **20**, 134–136.

Oates, M. (2000) Liaison psychiatry in the maternity hospital. In *Liaison Psychiatry: Planning Services for Specialist Settings* (eds R. Peveler, E. Feldman & T. Friedman), pp. 136–141. Gaskell.

Orrell, M. & Hancock, G. (2004) *The Camberwell Assessment of Need for the Elderly (CANE)*. Gaskell.

Oyserman, D., Bybee, D., Mowbray, C. T., *et al* (2004) Parenting self-construals of mothers with a serious mental illness: efficacy, burden and personal growth. *Journal of Applied Social Psychology*, **34**, 2503–2523.

Pachter, L. M., Auinger, P., Palmer, R., *et al* (2006) Do parenting and the home environment, maternal depression, neighbourhood and chronic poverty affect child behaviour problems differently in different racial-ethnic groups? *Pediatrics*, **117**, 1329–1338.

Pearlman, M. D., Tintinalli, J. E. & Lorenz, R. P. (1990) A prospective controlled study of outcome after trauma during pregnancy. *American Journal of Obstetric Gynecology*, **162**, 1502–1507.

Pfuhlmann, B., Stöber, G., Franzek, E., *et al* (1998) Cycloid psychoses predominate in severe postpartum psychiatric disorders. *Journal of Affective Disorders*, **50**, 125–134.

Phelan, M., Slade, M., Thornicroft, G., *et al* (1995) The Camberwell Assessment of Need: the validity and reliability of an instrument to assess the needs of people with severe mental illness. *British Journal of Psychiatry*, **167**, 589–595.

Poehlmann, J. & Fiese, B. H. (2001) The interaction of maternal and infant vulnerabilities on developing attachment relationships. *Development and Psychopathology*, **13**, 1–11.

Post, R. D., Willett, A. B., Franks, R. D., *et al* (1980) A preliminary report on the prevalence of domestic violence among psychiatric inpatients. *American Journal of Psychiatry*, **137**, 974–975.

Pryce, L. & Griffiths, R. (1993) How important is the assessment of social skills in current long-stay patients? *British Journal of Psychiatry*, **162**, 498–502.

Radke-Yarrow, M., Cummings, E. M., Kuczynski, L., *et al* (1985) Patterns of Attachment in two and three year olds in normal families and families with parental depression. *Child Development*, **56**, 884–893.

Radke-Yarrow, M., Nottelmann, E., Belmont, B., *et al* (1993) Affective interactions of depressed and nondepressed mothers and their children. *Journal of Abnormal Child Psychology*, **21**, 683–695.

Read, J., van Os, J., Morrison, A. P., *et al* (2005) Childhood trauma, psychosis and schizophrenia: a literature review with theoretical and clinical implications. *Acta Psychiatrica Scandinavica*, **112**, 330–350.

Reder, P. & Duncan, S. (1997) Adult psychiatry – a missing link in the child protection network: comments on Falcov's 'Fatal child abuse and parental psychiatric disorder'. *Child Abuse Review*, **6**, 35–40.

Reder, P. & Duncan, S. (1999) *Lost Innocents: A Follow Up Study of Fatal Child Abuse*. Routledge.

Renker, P. R. & Tonkin, P. (2006) Women's views of prenatal violence screening: acceptability and confidentiality issues. *Obstetrics and Gynecology*, **107**(2 Pt 1), 348–354.

Reynolds, T., Thornicroft, G., Abas, M., *et al* (2000) Camberwell Assessment of Need for the Elderly (CANE); development, validity, and reliability. *British Journal of Psychiatry*, **176**, 444–452.

Richman, N., Stevenson, J. & Graham, P. J. (1982) *Preschool to School: A Behavioural Study*. Academic Press.

Riordan, D., Appleby, L. & Faragher, B. (1999) Mother–infant interaction in post-partum women with schizophrenia and affective disorders. *Psychological Medicine*, **29**, 991–995.

Ritscher, J. E. B., Coursey, R. D., Farrell, E. W. (1997) A survey on issues in the lives of women with severe mental illness. *Psychiatric Services*, **48**, 1273–1282.

Rodnick, E. H. & Goldsein, M. J. (1974) Premorbid adjustment and the recovery of mothering function in acute schizophrenic women. *Journal of Abnormal Psychology*, **83**, 623–628.

Rodriguez, M. A., Ouiroga, S. S. & Bauer, H. M. (1996) Breaking the silence. Battered women's perspectives on medical care. *Archives of Family Medicine*, **5**, 153–158.

Rogosch, F. A., Mowbray, C. T. & Bogat, G. A. (1992) Determinants of parenting attitudes in mothers with severe psychopathology. *Development and Psychopathology*, **4**, 469–487.

Roy, R. (1990) Consequences of parental illness on children: a review. *Social Work and Social Sciences Review*, **2**, 109–121.

Roy, R., Neale, M. C., Pedersen, N. L., *et al* (1995) A twin study of generalised anxiety disorder and major depression. *Psychological Medicine*, **25**, 1037–1049.

Royal College of Psychiatrists (2002). *CR102. Domestic Violence*. Royal College of Psychiatrists.

Rudolph, B., Larson, G. L., Sweeney, S., *et al* (1990) Hospitalised pregnant women: characteristics and treatment issues. *Hospital and Community Psychiatry*, **41**, 159–163.

Rutter, M. (1966) *Children of Sick Parents: An Environmental and Psychiatric Study. Maudsley Monograph No 16*. Oxford University Press.

Rutter, M. (1982) Epidemiological-longitudinal approaches to the study of development. In *The Concept of Development: Minnesota Symposia on Child Psychology Vol. 15* (ed W. A. Collins): pp. 105–144. Lawrence Erlbaum.

Rutter, M. (1988) *Studies of Psychosocial Risk: The Power of Longitudinal Data*. Cambridge University Press.

Rutter, M. & Quinton, D. (1984) Parental psychiatric disorder: effects on children. *Psychological Medicine*, **14**, 853–880.

Rutter, M. & Silberg, J. (2002) Gene environment interplay in relation to emotional and behavioural disturbance. *Annual Review Psychology*, **53**, 463–490.

Rutter, M., MacDonald, H., Le Couteur, A., *et al*. (1990) Genetic factors in child psychiatric disorders – II Empirical findings. *Journal of Child Psychology and Psychiatry*, **31**, 39–83.

Sands, R. (1995) The parenting experience of low-income single women with serious mental disorders. *Families in Society*, **76**, 86–96.

Sands, R., Koppelman, N. & Solomon, P. (2004) Maternal custody status and living arrangements of children of women with severe mental illness. *Health and Social Work*, **29**, 317–325.

Savvidou, I., Vasilis, F., Hatzigeleki, S., *et al* (2003) Narratives about their children by mothers hospitalised on a psychiatric unit. *Family Process*, **42**, 391–402.

Seneviratne, G,. Conroy, S. & Marks, M. (2001) Parenting assessment in a psychiatric mother and baby unit. *Journal of Reproductive and Infant Psychology*, **19**, 274.

Shah, N. & Howard, L.M. (2006) Screening for smoking and substance misuse in pregnant women with mental illness. *Psychiatric Bulletin*, **30**, 294–297.

Sharp, D., Hay, D. F., Pawlby, S., *et al* (1995) The impact of post-natal depression on boys' intellectual development. *Journal of Child Psychology and Psychiatry*, **36**, 1315–1337.

Silberg, J., Rutter, M., Neale, M., *et al* (2001) Genetic moderation of environmental risk for depression and anxiety in adolescent girls. *British Journal of Psychiatry*, **179**, 116–121.

Slade, M. (2002) Routine outcome assessment in mental health services. *Psychological Medicine*, **32**, 1339–1344.

Slade, M. & Glover, G. (2001) The needs of people with mental disorders. In *Textbook of Community Psychiatry* (eds G. Thornicroft & G. Szmukler): pp. 117–127. Oxford University Press.

Slade, M., Loftus, L., Phelan, M., *et al* (1999*a*) *The Camberwell Assessment of Need*. Gaskell.

Slade, M., Leese, M., Taylor, R., *et al* (1999*b*) The association between needs and quality of life in an epidemiologically representative sample of people with psychosis. *Acta Psychiatrica Scandinavica*, **100**, 149–157.

Slade, M., Powell, R., Rosen, A., *et al* (2000) Threshold Assessment Grid (TAG): The development of a valid and brief scale to assess the severity of mental illness. *Social Psychiatry and Psychiatric Epidemiology*, **35**, 78–85.

Slade, M., Leese, M., Ruggeri, M., *et al* (2004) Does meeting needs improve quality of life? *Psychotherapy and Psychosomatics*, **73**, 183–189.

Slade, M., Leese, M., Cahill, S., *et al* (2005) Patient-rated mental health needs and quality of life improvement. *British Journal of Psychiatry*, **187**, 256–261.

Slade, M., McCrone, P., Kuipers, E., *et al* (2006) Use of standardised outcome measures in adult mental health services: randomised controlled trial. *British Journal of Psychiatry*, **189**, 330–336.

Smith, M. (2004) Parental mental health: disruptions to parenting and outcomes for children. *Child and Family Social Work*, **9**, 3–11.

Solantaus-Simula, T., Punamaki, R. L. & Beardslee, W. R. (2002) Children's responses to low parental mood. 1: Balancing between active empathy, overinvolvment, indifference and avoidance. *Journal of the American Academy of Child and Adolescent Psychiatry*, **41**, 278–286.

Spielvogel, A. & Wile, J. (1992) Treatment and outcomes of psychotic patients during pregnancy and childbirth. *Birth*, **19**, 131–137.

Stallard, P., Norman, D. K., Huline-Dickens, S., *et al* (2004) The effects of parental mental illness upon children: a descriptive study of the views of parents and children. *Clinical Child Psychology and Psychiatry*, **9**, 39–52.

Steichen, T. J. & Cox, N. J. (2002) A note on the concordance correlation coefficient. *The Stata Journal*, **2**, 183–189.

Stein, A., Gath, D. H., Bucher, J., *et al* (1991) The relationship between parental depression and mother–child interactions. *British Journal of Psychiatry*, **158**, 46–52.

Stevens, A. & Gabbay, J. (1991) Needs assessment needs assessment. *Health Trends*, **23**, 20–23.

Stewart, D. & Gangbar, R. (1984) Psychiatric assessment of competency to care for a newborn. *Canadian Journal of Psychiatry*, **29**, 583–589.

Taylor, C. G., Norman, D. K., Murphy, J. M., *et al* (1991) Diagnosed intellectual and emotional impairment among parents who seriously mistreat their children: prevalence, type and outcome in a court sample. *Child Abuse and Neglect*, **15**, 389–401.

Taylor, E. (1991) Developmental neuropsychiatry. *Journal of Child Psychology and Psychiatry*, **32**, 1–48.

Terp, I. M. & Mortensen, P. B. (1998) Post-partum psychoses. Clinical diagnoses and relative risk of admission after parturition. *British Journal of Psychiatry*, **172**, 521–526.

Thomas, S., Harty, M., Parrott, J., *et al* (2003) *The Forensic CAN: Camberwell Assessment of Need Forensic Version (CANFOR)*. Gaskell.

Thomas, S., Slade, M., McCrone, P., *et al* (2008) The reliability and validity of the Forensic Camberwell Assessment of Need (CANFOR): a needs assessment for forensic mental health service users. *International Journal of Methods in Psychiatric Research*, 2008, in press.

Thompson, S. & Pudney, S. (1990) *Mental Illness: The Fundamental Facts*. Mental Health Foundation.

Thornicroft, G. (2006) *Shunned. Discrimination Against People with Mental Illness*. Oxford University Press.

Tienari, P., Wynne, L. C., Moring, J., *et al* (1994) The Finnish Adoptive Family Study of schizophrenia: implications for family research. *British Journal of Psychiatry*, **164** (suppl 23), 20–26.

Trixler, M., Gati, A., Fekete, S., *et al* (2005) Use of antipsychotics in the management of schizophrenia during pregnancy. *Drugs*, **65**, 1193–1206.

UK700 Group (1999) Predictors of quality of life in people with severe mental illness. Study methodology with baseline analysis in the UK700 trial. *British Journal of Psychiatry*, **175**, 426–432.

van Haaster, I., LeSage, A., Cyr, M., *et al* (1994) Problems and needs for care of patients suffering from severe mental illness. *Social Psychiatry and Psychiatric Epidemiology*, **29**, 141–148.

van Os, J., Altamura, A. C., Bobes, J., *et al* (2004) Evaluation of the Two-Way Communication Checklist as a clinical intervention. *British Journal of Psychiatry*, **184**, 79–83.

Viguera, A. C., Nonacs, R., Cohen, L. S., *et al* (2000) Risk of recurrence of bipolar disorder in pregnant and nonpregnant women after discontinuing lithium maintenance. *American Journal of Psychiatry*, **157**, 179–184.

Walsh, C., MacMillan, H. & Jamieson, E. (2002) The relationship between parental psychiatric disorder and child physical and sexual abuse: findings from the Ontario Health Supplement. *Child Abuse and Neglect*, **26**, 11–22.

Wang, A. R. & Goldschmidt, V. V. (1994) Interviews of psychiatric inpatients about their family situation and young children. *Acta Psychiatrica Scandinavica*, **90**, 459–465.

Wang, A. R. & Goldschmidt, V. V. (1996) Interviews with psychiatric inpatients about professional intervention with regard to their children. *Acta Psychiatrica Scandinavica*, **93**, 57–61.

Watts, C. & Zimmerman, C. (2002) Violence against women: global scope and magnitude. *Lancet*, **359**, 1232–1237.

Webb, R. T., Howard, L. & Abel, K. M. (2004) Antipsychotic drugs for non-affective psychosis during pregnancy and postpartum. In *The Cochrane Library (Issue 2)*. Update Software.

Webb, R., Abel, K., Pickles, A., et al (2005) Mortality in offspring of parents with psychotic disorders: a critical review and meta-analysis. *American Journal of Psychiatry*, **162**, 1045–1056.

Webb, R. T., Abel, K. M., Pickles, A. R., et al (2006). Mortality risk among offspring of psychiatric inpatients: a population-based follow-up to early adulthood. *American Journal of Psychiatry*, **163**, 2170–2177.

Weinberg, M. K. & Tronick, E. Z. (1998) Emotional characteristics of infants associated with maternal depression and anxiety. *Pediatrics*, **102**(5, suppl E), 1298–1304.

Weissman, M. M., Feder, A., Pilowsky, D. J., et al (2004) Depressed mothers coming to primary care: Maternal reports of problems with their children. *Journal of Affective Disorders*, **78**, 93–100.

Weissman, M. M., Wickramaratne, P. J., Nomura, Y., et al (2005) Families at high and low risk for depression: a three-generation study. *Archives of General Psychiatry*, **62**, 29–36.

Weissman, M. M., Wickramaratne, P., Nomura, Y., et al (2006a) Offspring of depressed parents: 20 years later. *American Journal of Psychiatry*, **163**, 1001–1008.

Weissman, M. M., Pilowsky, D. J., Wickramaratne, P. J., et al (2006b) Remissions in maternal depression and child psychopathology: a STAR*D-child report. *JAMA*, **295**, 1389–1398.

Whitaker, R. C., Orzol, S. M. & Kahn, R. S. (2006) Maternal mental health, substance use, and domestic violence in the year after delivery and subsequent behaviour problems in children at age 3 years. *Archives of General Psychiatry*, **63**, 551–560.

White, C. L., Nicholson, J., Fisher, W. H., et al (1995) Mothers with severe mental illness caring for children. *Journal of Nervous and Mental Disease*, **183**, 398–403.

Wiersma, D., Nienhuis, F. J., Giel, R., et al (1998) Stability and change in needs of patients with schizophrenic disorders: a 15- and 17-year follow-up from first onset of psychosis, and a comparison between 'objective' and 'subjective' assessments of needs for care. *Social Psychiatry and Psychiatric Epidemiology*, **33**, 49–56.

Wilczynski, A. (1994) The incidence of child homicide: how accurate are the official statistics? *Journal of Clinical Forensic Medicine*, **1**, 61–66.

Wilczynski, A. (1995) Risk factors for parental child homicide: results of an English study. *Current Issues in Criminal Justice*, **7**, 241–253.

Wiseman, M. & Lewis, S. (2006) Getting it right when things go wrong: an analysis of serious case reviews occurring in a mental health trust. Paper presented at XVIth ISPCAN International Congress on Child Abuse and Neglect, York, UK.

Wolfe, D. A., Crookes, C. V., Lee, V., et al (2003) The effects of children's exposure to domestic violence: a meta-analysis and critique. *Clinical Child and Family Psychology Reviews*, **6**, 171–187.

Wrede, G,. Mednick, S. A., Huttunen, M. O., et al (1980) Pregnancy and delivery complications in the births of an unselected series of Finnish children with schizophrenic mothers. *Acta Psychiatrica Scandinavica*, **62**, 369–381.

Xenitidis, K., Thornicroft, G., Leese, M., et al (2000) Reliability and validity of CANDID – a needs assessment instrument for adults with learning disabilities and mental health problems. *British Journal of Psychiatry*, **176**, 473–478.

Xenitidis, K., Slade, M., Bouras, N., et al (2003) *CANDID: Camberwell Assessment of Need for adults with Developmental and Intellectual Disabilities*. Gaskell.

Zankowski, G. L. (1987) Responsive programming: meeting the needs of chemically dependent women. *Alcoholism Treatment Quarterly*, **4**, 53–66.

Zeitlin, D., Dhanjal, T., Colmsee, M. (1999) Maternal-foetal bonding: the impact of domestic violence on the bonding process between a mother and a child. *Archives of Women's Mental Health*, **2**, 183–189.

Zeitlin, H. (1986) *The Natural History of Disorder in Childhood*. Oxford University Press.

Zuravin, S. J. (1988) Child abuse, child neglect, and maternal depression: is there a connection? In *Child Neglect Monograph: Proceedings from a Symposium*. Office of Human Development Services Washington DC.

# Index

# Appendix 1

## Coversheet for all versions of the Camberwell Assessment of Need for Mothers (CAN–M)

# Camberwell Assessment of Need for Mothers (CAN–M)

Assessment date: _____ / _____ / _____
User name/ID: _____
Interviewer: _____

## Child protection issues to consider

When completing the CAN–M questionnaire please give consideration to the impact of the mother's state on the child at all times, especially when unmet needs, or moderate or high help, has been identified in the domains of *Self-care* (4), *Psychotic symptoms* (9), *Psychological distress* (10), *Safety to self* (12), *Safety to child/children and others* (13), *Substance misuse* (14), *Violence and abuse* (18), *Practical demands of childcare* (19), and the *Emotional demands of childcare* (20). If you identify concerns about the impact on the child, then please discuss these concerns with your supervisor or manager. If, after this discussion, you still have concerns and feel that the child and mother would benefit from further services, please speak to the mother's care coordinator. If you consider the child is at suspected or identified risk, however, refer to your local social services.

## Coversheet

(1) Service user

(i) Name: _____ (ii) Date of birth: _____ / _____ / _____

(iii) Contact details:

Address: _____

Home phone: _____ Mobile: _____

(2) Dependants

(i) Is the service user pregnant? Yes / No (please circle correct answer)

(ii) If yes, is the service user attending regular antenatal appointments? Yes / No (please give details)
_____
_____
_____

(iii) Number of children (under the age of 16 years):

(iv) Age and sex of child/children (youngest to eldest):

Child 1: Age ☐ Sex ☐          Child 3: Age ☐ Sex ☐          Child 5: Age ☐ Sex ☐

Child 2: Age ☐ Sex ☐          Child 4: Age ☐ Sex ☐          Child 6: Age ☐ Sex ☐

(v) Living arrangements of child/children (you may tick more than one option):

Mother ☐                Friend ☐                        Children's home ☐        Relatives ☐
Father (if separated) ☐  Foster family (unrelated) ☐      Adopted ☐

(3) Care coordinator

(i) Name: _____ (ii) Title / position: _____

(iii) Contact details: _____

# Appendix 2

# Camberwell Assessment of Need for Mothers (Clinical version) – CAN–M (C)

# Camberwell Assessment of Need for Mothers (CAN–M)

Assessment date: _____ / _____ / _____

User name/ID: _____

Interviewer: _____

## Child protection issues to consider

When completing the CAN–M questionnaire please give consideration to the impact of the mother's state on the child at all times, especially when unmet needs, or moderate or high help, has been identified in the domains of *Self-care* (4), *Psychotic symptoms* (9), *Psychological distress* (10), *Safety to self* (12), *Safety to child/children and others* (13), *Substance misuse* (14), *Violence and abuse* (18), *Practical demands of childcare* (19), and the *Emotional demands of childcare* (20). If you identify concerns about the impact on the child, then please discuss these concerns with your supervisor or manager. If, after this discussion, you still have concerns and feel that the child and mother would benefit from further services, please speak to the mother's care coordinator. If you consider the child is at suspected or identified risk, however, refer to your local social services.

## Coversheet

(1) Service user

(i) Name: _____ (ii) Date of birth: _____ / _____ / _____

(iii) Contact details:

Address: _____

Home phone: _____ Mobile: _____

(2) Dependants

(i) Is the service user pregnant? Yes / No (please circle correct answer)

(ii) If yes, is the service user attending regular antenatal appointments? Yes / No
(please give details)

_____

_____

_____

(iii) Number of children (under the age of 16 years):

(iv) Age and sex of child/children (youngest to eldest):

Child 1: Age [___] Sex [___]     Child 3: Age [___] Sex [___]     Child 5: Age [___] Sex [___]

Child 2: Age [___] Sex [___]     Child 4: Age [___] Sex [___]     Child 6: Age [___] Sex [___]

(v) Living arrangements of child/children (you may tick more than one option):

Mother ☐     Friend ☐     Children's home ☐     Relatives ☐

Father (if separated) ☐     Foster family (unrelated) ☐     Adopted ☐

(3) Care coordinator

(i) Name: _____ (ii) Title / position: _____

(iii) Contact details: _____

# 1 Accomodation

Assessments

User   Staff

### Does the person have an appropriate place to live now or following hospital discharge?

*Is your current accommodation appropriate?*

*(If in hospital) Do you have a place to live?*

| Rating | Meaning | Example |
|---|---|---|
| 0 | No need | Accommodation is adequate, secure and childsafe (e.g. child locks, safety gates) |
| 1 | Met need | Person has adequate supported accommodation |
| 2 | Unmet need | Home lacks basic facilities such as water and electricity |
| 9 | Not known | |

*If rated 0 or 9 go to Question 2*

### How much help with accommodation does the person receive from partner, friends or relatives?

| Rating | Meaning | Example |
|---|---|---|
| 0 | None | |
| 1 | Low help | Advice and support |
| 2 | Moderate help | Would provide help with improving accommodation, providing furniture or redecoration |
| 3 | High help | Living with friend/family because own accommodation is unsatisfactory. |
| 9 | Not known | |

### How much help with accommodation does the person receive from local services?

### How much help with accommodation will the person need from local services?

| Rating | Meaning | Example |
|---|---|---|
| 0 | None | |
| 1 | Low help | Advice and support |
| 2 | Moderate help | Referral to housing agency for improvements or independent living |
| 3 | High help | Being rehoused, living in group home or hostel |
| 9 | Not known | |

### User's view of services required

| Action(s) | By whom | Review date |
|---|---|---|
| | | |

# 2 Food

### Does the person have difficulty in buying and preparing food?

*Are you able to prepare appropriate meals?*

*Are you able to do your own shopping?*

| Rating | Meaning | Example |
|---|---|---|
| 0 | No need | Able to buy and prepare appropriate meals |
| 1 | Met need | Requires assistance to buy or prepare appropriate food, or receives meals |
| 2 | Unmet need | Unable to buy or prepare food or not receiving appropriate help. Diet very limited |
| 9 | Not known | |

*If rated 0 or 9 go to Question 3*

### How much help does the person receive from partner, friends or relatives with buying and preparing food?

| Rating | Meaning | Example |
|---|---|---|
| 0 | None | |
| 1 | Low help | Requires nutritional advice. Weekly prompting or assistance with shopping or food preparation |
| 2 | Moderate help | Daily prompting or assistance with shopping or food preparation |
| 3 | High help | Meals provided daily |
| 9 | Not known | |

### How much help does the person receive from local services with buying and preparing food?

### How much help does the person need from local services with buying and preparing food?

| Rating | Meaning | Example |
|---|---|---|
| 0 | None | |
| 1 | Low help | Requires nutritional advice. Weekly prompting or assistance with shopping or food preparation |
| 2 | Moderate help | Daily prompting or assistance with shopping or food preparation. Attends cooking groups |
| 3 | High help | Meals provided daily |
| 9 | Not known | |

### User's view of services required

| Action(s) | By whom | Review date |
|---|---|---|
| | | |

# 3 Looking after the home

### Does the person have difficulty looking after her home?

*Are you able to look after your home or room?*

*Does anyone help you to keep your home/room tidy?*

| Rating | Meaning | Example |
|---|---|---|
| 0 | No need | Keeps home clean and tidy |
| 1 | Met need | Receives and needs regular domestic help |
| 2 | Unmet need | Home is dirty and a potential health hazard |
| 9 | Not known | |

*If rated 0 or 9 go to Question 4*

### How much help does the person receive from partner, friends or relatives with looking after her home?

| Rating | Meaning | Example |
|---|---|---|
| 0 | None | |
| 1 | Low help | Prompts or helps tidy-up occasionally |
| 2 | Moderate help | Prompts or helps clean at least once a week |
| 3 | High help | Supervises the person more than once a week, washes all clothes and cleans the home |
| 9 | Not known | |

### How much help does the person receive from local services with looking after her home?

### How much help does the person need from local services with looking after her home?

| Rating | Meaning | Example |
|---|---|---|
| 0 | None | |
| 1 | Low help | Occasional prompting or assistance by staff |
| 2 | Moderate help | Prompting or assistance at least once a week |
| 3 | High help | Majority of domestic tasks done by staff |
| 9 | Not known | |

### User's view of services required

| Action(s) | By whom | Review date |
|---|---|---|
| | | |

# 4 Self-care

### Does the person have difficulty with self-care?

*Do you have problems keeping clean and tidy?*

*Do you ever need reminding? Who by?*

| Rating | Meaning | Example |
|---|---|---|
| 0 | No need | Appearance may be unusual, eccentric or untidy, but is basically clean |
| 1 | Met need | Needs and gets help with self-care |
| 2 | Unmet need (consider impact on child) | Poor personel hygiene |
| 9 | Not known | |

*If rated 0 or 9 go to Question 5*

### How much help does the person receive from partner, friends or relatives with self-care?

| Rating | Meaning | Example |
|---|---|---|
| 0 | None | |
| 1 | Low help | Occasionally prompts person to change her clothes, brush her teeth, etc. |
| 2 | Moderate help | Run the bath/shower and insist on its use, daily prompting |
| 3 | High help | Daily assistance with several aspects of self-care |
| 9 | Not known | |

### How much help does the person receive from local services with self-care?

### How much help will the person need from local services with self-care?

| Rating | Meaning | Example |
|---|---|---|
| 0 | None | |
| 1 | Low help | Occasional prompting |
| 2 | Moderate help | Supervise self-care activities |
| 3 | High help | Physically assists with several aspects of self-care or self-care skills programme |
| 9 | Not known | |

### User's view of services required

| Action(s) | By whom | Review date |
|---|---|---|
| | | |

# 5 Daytime activities

## Does the person have difficulty with regular daytime activities?

*How do you spend your day?*

*Do you have enough to do during the day?*

| Rating | Meaning | Example |
|---|---|---|
| 0 | No need | Able to occupy self with work, household, social or childcare activities |
| 1 | Met need | Unable to occupy self, attending occupational therapy or day centre |
| 2 | Unmet need | Not adequately occupied with daytime activities |
| 9 | Not known | |

*If rated 0 or 9 go to Question 6*

## How much help does the person receive from partner, friends or relatives in finding or keeping regular daytime activities?

| Rating | Meaning | Example |
|---|---|---|
| 0 | None | |
| 1 | Low help | Occasional advice about daytime activities |
| 2 | Moderate help | Accompanied to leisure activities |
| 3 | High help | Daily help with arranging daytime activities |
| 9 | Not known | |

## How much help does the person receive from local services in finding or keeping regular daytime activities?

## How much help does the person need from local services in finding or keeping regular daytime activities?

| Rating | Meaning | Example |
|---|---|---|
| 0 | None | |
| 1 | Low help | Advice and information about activities and local facilities |
| 2 | Moderate help | Sheltered employment daily. Attends occupational therapy activities or day centre 2–4 days per week |
| 3 | High help | All daytime activities arranged by staff |
| 9 | Not known | |

## User's view of services required

| Action(s) | By whom | Review date |
|---|---|---|
| | | |

# 6 General physical health

Assessments

User   Staff

### Does the person have any general physical illness, disability or medication side-effects?

*How do you feel physically?*

*Are you getting treatment for physical problems from your doctor?*

| Rating | Meaning | Example |
|--------|---------|---------|
| 0 | No need | Physically well |
| 1 | Met need | Physical ailment, such as high blood pressure, receiving appropriate treatment |
| 2 | Unmet need | Untreated physical problems, including medication side-effects or ineffective treatment |
| 9 | Not known | |

*If rated 0 or 9 go to Question 7*

### How much help does the person receive from partner, friends or relatives for general physical problems?

| Rating | Meaning | Example |
|--------|---------|---------|
| 0 | None | |
| 1 | Low help | Prompting to see a doctor |
| 2 | Moderate help | Accompanied to medical appointments |
| 3 | High help | Daily help with going to the toilet, eating or mobility |
| 9 | Not known | |

### How much help does the person receive from local services for general physical problems?

### How much help does the person need from local services for general physical problems?

| Rating | Meaning | Example |
|--------|---------|---------|
| 0 | None | |
| 1 | Low help | Given general health advice |
| 2 | Moderate help | Regular review/involvement of specialist medical services (e.g. dietician, GP). Prescribed medication |
| 3 | High help | In-patient or frequent hospital appointments. Alterations to home |
| 9 | Not known | |

### User's view of services required

| Action(s) | By whom | Review date |
|-----------|---------|-------------|
| | | |

# 7 Pregnancy care

## Does the person have any physical problems relating to pregnancy or after the birth?

*Do you have any physical problems with your pregnancy?*

*Did you have any birth complications?*

*Are you attending your antenatal appointments?*

| Rating | Meaning | Example |
|---|---|---|
| 0 | No need | Fully recovered from pregnancy and birth |
| 1 | Met need | Receiving appropriate care and monitoring. Attending regular antenatal appointments |
| 2 | Unmet need | Untreated physical problems, including medication side-effects, ineffective treatment or poor antenatal/postnatal care |
| 8 | Not applicable (user is not pregnant or has not recently given birth) | |
| 9 | Not known | |

*If rated 0 or 9 go to Question 8*

## How much help does the person receive from partner, friends or relatives for physical problems relating to pregnancy care?

| Rating | Meaning | Example |
|---|---|---|
| 0 | None | |
| 1 | Low help | Prompting to attend antenatal check-ups |
| 2 | Moderate help | Accompanied to medical appointments |
| 3 | High help | Daily help required owing to physical problems |
| 9 | Not known | |

## How much help does the person receive from local services for physical problems relating to pregnancy care?

## How much help does the person need from local services for problems relating to pregnancy care?

| Rating | Meaning | Example |
|---|---|---|
| 0 | None | |
| 1 | Low help | Given health advice, including dietary advice and breastfeeding information |
| 2 | Moderate help | Involvement of specialist medical services |
| 3 | High help | In-patient or frequent hospital appointments |
| 9 | Not known | |

## User's view of services required

| Action(s) | By whom | Review date |
|---|---|---|
| | | |

# 8 Sleep

### Does the person have any problems with her sleep?

*How well are you sleeping?*

| Rating | Meaning | Example |
|--------|---------|---------|
| 0 | No need | Gets adequate sleep |
| 1 | Met need | Uses sleep aids such as relaxation exercises or music. Shares childcare responsibilities at night |
| 2 | Unmet need | Severely disrupted sleep. Regularly has less than 4 hours per night or unrefreshing sleep |
| 9 | Not known | |

*If rated 0 or 9 go to Question 9*

### How much help does the person receive from partner, friends or relatives for problems with sleep?

| Rating | Meaning | Example |
|--------|---------|---------|
| 0 | None | |
| 1 | Low help | Advice, sympathy and suppport |
| 2 | Moderate help | Prompts the use of sleeping aids. Shares childcare responsibilities at night |
| 3 | High help | Assistance with sleep programme. Family and friends care for child at night |
| 9 | Not known | |

### How much help does the person receive from local services for problems with sleep?

### How much help does the person need from local services for problems with sleep?

| Rating | Meaning | Example |
|--------|---------|---------|
| 0 | None | |
| 1 | Low help | Sleep education |
| 2 | Moderate help | Sleep programme such as the 'controlled crying' technique |
| 3 | High help | Referral to sleep centre, prescribed medication. Hospital staff care for child at night |
| 9 | Not known | |

### User's view of services required

| Action(s) | By whom | Review date |
|-----------|---------|-------------|
| | | |

# 9  Psychotic symptoms

## Does the person have any psychotic symptoms such as hallucinations or delusional beliefs?

*Do you ever hear voices or have problems with your thoughts?*

*Are you on medication or injections? What is it for?*

| Rating | Meaning | Example |
|---|---|---|
| 0 | No need | No positive symptoms, not at risk from symptoms and not on medication |
| 1 | Met need | Symptoms helped by medication or other treatment, e.g. psychological therapy |
| 2 | Unmet need (consider impact on child) | Untreated psychosis/postnatal psychosis or at high risk of relapse |
| 9 | Not known | |

*If rated 0 or 9 go to Question 10*

## How much help does the person receive from partner, friends or relatives for these psychotic symptoms?

| Rating | Meaning | Example |
|---|---|---|
| 0 | None | |
| 1 | Low help | Sympathy and support |
| 2 | Moderate help | Carers involved in helping with coping strategies, relapse prevention and/or medication compliance |
| 3 | High help | Constant supervision of medication, coping strategies and relapse prevention |
| 9 | Not known | |

## How much help does the person receive from local services for these psychotic symptoms?

## How much help does the person need from local services for these psychotic symptoms?

| Rating | Meaning | Example |
|---|---|---|
| 0 | None | |
| 1 | Low help | Maintenance of medication |
| 2 | Moderate help | Regular review of medication and care plan. Attends support groups or psychotherapy |
| 3 | High help | Medication and 24-hour hospital care or crisis care at home |
| 9 | Not known | |

## User's view of services required

| Action(s) | By whom | Review date |
|---|---|---|
| | | |

# 10 Psychological distress

### Does the person suffer from current psychological distress, anxiety or depression?

*Have you recently felt sad or low?*

*Have you felt overly anxious or frightened?*

*Has your mood changed since giving birth?*

| Rating | Meaning | Example |
|---|---|---|
| 0 | No need | Occasional or mild distress |
| 1 | Met need | Needs and receives ongoing support |
| 2 | Unmet need (consider impact on child) | Has expressed suicidal ideas during the last month or has exposed themselves to serious danger |
| 9 | Not known | |

*If rated 0 or 9 go to Question 11*

### How much help does the person receive from partner, friends or relatives for this distress?

| Rating | Meaning | Example |
|---|---|---|
| 0 | None | |
| 1 | Low help | Some sympathy and support |
| 2 | Moderate help | Opportunity at least weekly to talk about distress to friend or relative |
| 3 | High help | Constant support and supervision |
| 9 | Not known | |

### How much help does the person receive from local services for this distress?
### How much help does the person need from local services for this distress?

| Rating | Meaning | Example |
|---|---|---|
| 0 | None | |
| 1 | Low help | Assessment of mental state or occasional support |
| 2 | Moderate help | Specific psychological or social treatment. Counselled by staff at least once a week |
| 3 | High help | 24-hour hospital care or crisis care |
| 9 | Not known | |

### User's view of services required

| Action(s) | By whom | Review date |
|---|---|---|
| | | |

# 11 Information

## Has the person had clear verbal or written information about her condition, care plan and rights?

*Have you been given clear information about your condition and treatment?*

*Do you understand the role of each professional in your treatment?*

*(Where relevant) Do you know your rights under the Mental Health Act?*

| Rating | Meaning | Example |
|--------|---------|---------|
| 0 | No need | Information retained from previous contact with local services |
| 1 | Met need | Has received and understands sufficient information |
| 2 | Unmet need | Has not received or fails to understand sufficient information. Absence of care plan or pre-birth conference |
| 9 | Not known | |

*If rated 0 or 9 go to Question 12*

## How much help does the person receive from partner, friends or relatives in obtaining such information?

| Rating | Meaning | Example |
|--------|---------|---------|
| 0 | None | |
| 1 | Low help | Some advice given |
| 2 | Moderate help | Given leaflets or put in touch with self-help groups |
| 3 | High help | Regular liaison with doctors or local support groups |
| 9 | Not known | |

## How much help does the person receive from local services in obtaining such information?

## How much help does the person need from local services in obtaining such information?

| Rating | Meaning | Example |
|--------|---------|---------|
| 0 | None | |
| 1 | Low help | Brief verbal or written information |
| 2 | Moderate help | Informal discussions with staff on a range of issues relevant to condition and treatment |
| 3 | High help | Regular structured information sessions with staff to improve knowledge and understanding of condition and treatment |
| 9 | Not known | |

## User's view of services required

| Action(s) | By whom | Review date |
|-----------|---------|-------------|
|           |         |             |

# 12 Safety to self

### Is the person a danger to herself

☐ ☐

*Do you ever have thoughts of harming yourself?*

*Have you harmed yourself recently?*

*Do you put yourself in danger in any way?*

| Rating | Meaning | Example |
|--------|---------|---------|
| 0 | No need | No thoughts of suicide or self-harm |
| 1 | Met need | Risk identified and monitored by staff, receiving counselling |
| 2 | Unmet need (consider impact on child) | Has expressed or acted out suicidal ideas, has exposed self to serious danger |
| 9 | Not known | |

*If rated 0 or 9 go to Question 13*

### How much help does the person receive from partner, friends or relatives to reduce the risk of self-harm?

☐ ☐

| Rating | Meaning | Example |
|--------|---------|---------|
| 0 | None | |
| 1 | Low help | Able to contact friends or relatives if feeling unsafe |
| 2 | Moderate help | Friends or relatives are usually in contact and are likely to know if person is feeling unsafe |
| 3 | High help | Friends or relatives are in regular contact and would inform staff if disclosed/suspected risk |
| 9 | Not known | |

### How much help does the person receive from local services to reduce the risk of self-harm?

☐ ☐

### How much help does the person need from local services to reduce the risk of self-harm?

☐ ☐

| Rating | Meaning | Example |
|--------|---------|---------|
| 0 | None | |
| 1 | Low help | Someone to contact if feeling unsafe |
| 2 | Moderate help | Staff check at least once a week, receiving supportive counselling |
| 3 | High help | Daily supervision, in-patient care |
| 9 | Not known | |

### User's view of services required

| Action(s) | By whom | Review date |
|-----------|---------|-------------|
| | | |

# 13 Safety to child/children and others

Assessments

User    Staff

## Is the person a current or potential risk to her child/children's safety or to other people's safety?

*Do you think you could be a danger to other people's safety?*

*Have you threatened other people or been violent?*

*Do you ever lose your temper and hit your child/children?*

| Rating | Meaning | Example |
|---|---|---|
| 0 | No need | No history of violence or threatening behaviour |
| 1 | Met need | Monitoring risk, receives sufficient appropriate help for this problem |
| 2 | Unmet need (consider impact on child) | Recent harm, violence, threatening behaviour or neglect |
| 9 | Not known | |

*If rated 0 or 9 go to Question 14*

## How much help does the person receive from partner, friends or relatives to reduce the risk that she might harm someone else?

| Rating | Meaning | Example |
|---|---|---|
| 0 | None | |
| 1 | Low help | General advice about threatening behaviour |
| 2 | Moderate help | Support/supervision more than weekly |
| 3 | High help | Daily support/supervision |
| 9 | Not known | |

## How much help does the person receive from local services to reduce the risk that she might harm someone else?

## How much help does the person need from local services to reduce the risk that she might harm someone else?

| Rating | Meaning | Example |
|---|---|---|
| 0 | None | |
| 1 | Low help | Check on behaviour monthly or less, general advice and support |
| 2 | Moderate help | Regular check-ups on behaviour. referral to social services |
| 3 | High help | Constant supervision. Intensive parenting programme. Child removed |
| 9 | Not known | |

## User's view of services required

| Action(s) | By whom | Review date |
|---|---|---|
| | | |

# 14 Substance misuse

## Does the person have problems with alcohol or drug misuse?

*Does drinking cause you problems?*

*Do you take any drugs that are not prescribed by a doctor?*

*Do you find it difficult to stop?*

| Rating | Meaning | Example |
|---|---|---|
| 0 | No need | No alcohol or drug problem |
| 1 | Met need | At risk from substance misuse and receiving help |
| 2 | Unmet need (consider impact on child) | Harmful and/or uncontrolled use |
| 9 | Not known | |

*If rated 0 or 9 go to Question 15*

## How much help does the person receive from partner, friends or relatives for their substance misuse?

| Rating | Meaning | Example |
|---|---|---|
| 0 | None | |
| 1 | Low help | Encouraged to reduce substance intake |
| 2 | Moderate help | Regular advice, put in contact with helping agencies |
| 3 | High help | Reported concerns to clinical team, working in partnership to reduce intake |
| 9 | Not known | |

## How much help does the person receive from local services for their substance misuse?

## How much help does the person need from local services for their substance misuse?

| Rating | Meaning | Example |
|---|---|---|
| 0 | None | |
| 1 | Low help | Informed about risks, given leaflets |
| 2 | Moderate help | Given details of helping agencies. Counselling |
| 3 | High help | Attends specialist clinic. Supervised withdrawal programme |
| 9 | Not known | |

## User's view of services required

| Action(s) | By whom | Review date |
|---|---|---|
| | | |

# 15 Company

## Does the person need help with social contact?

*Are you happy with your social life?*

*Do you wish you had more contact with others?*

| Rating | Meaning | Example |
|---|---|---|
| 0 | No need | Able to organise social contact, has enough friends or content with own company |
| 1 | Met need | Attends organised social events, frequently accompanied by support person |
| 2 | Unmet need | Frequently feels lonely and isolated |
| 9 | Not known | |

*If rated 0 or 9 go to Question 16*

## How much help with social contact does the person receive from partner, friends or relatives?

| Rating | Meaning | Example |
|---|---|---|
| 0 | None | |
| 1 | Low help | Social contact less than weekly |
| 2 | Moderate help | Social contact weekly or more often |
| 3 | High help | Social contact at least four times a week |
| 9 | Not known | |

## How much help with social contact does the person receive from local services?

## How much help with social contact does the person need from local services?

| Rating | Meaning | Example |
|---|---|---|
| 0 | None | |
| 1 | Low help | Encourages participation in social activities |
| 2 | Moderate help | Given advice about social clubs or social skills groups |
| 3 | High help | Attends day centre or community group |
| 9 | Not known | |

## User's view of services required

| Action(s) | By whom | Review date |
|---|---|---|
| | | |

# 16 Intimate relationships

## Does the person have any difficulty in starting or maintaining a close relationship?

*Do you have a partner?*

*Do you have problems in your partnership/marriage?*

| Rating | Meaning | Example |
|---|---|---|
| 0 | No need | Satisfactory relationship or content not having a partner |
| 1 | Met need | Receiving helpful advice or therapy |
| 2 | Unmet need | Wants a partner and feels not having one is a problem or unhappy in existing relationship |
| 9 | Not known | |

*If rated 0 or 9 go to Question 17*

## How much help does the person receive from partner, friends or relatives with starting and maintaining close relationships?

| Rating | Meaning | Example |
|---|---|---|
| 0 | None | |
| 1 | Low help | Some support |
| 2 | Moderate help | Regular support and advice. Prompts use of self-help books, etc. |
| 3 | High help | Intensive support in coping with feelings |
| 9 | Not known | |

## How much help does the person receive from local services with starting and maintaining close relationships?

## How much help does the person need from local services with starting and maintaining close relationships?

| Rating | Meaning | Example |
|---|---|---|
| 0 | None | |
| 1 | Low help | Some relationship support |
| 2 | Moderate help | Regular relationship support and advice. Prompts use of self-help books, etc. |
| 3 | High help | Therapy, social skills training |
| 9 | Not known | |

## User's view of services required

| Action(s) | By whom | Review date |
|---|---|---|
| | | |

# 17 Sexual health

### Does the person have problems with her sex life?

*How is your sex life?*

*Do you require information about safe sex or contraception?*

| Rating | Meaning | Example |
|---|---|---|
| 0 | No need | Content with sex life |
| 1 | Met need | Benefiting from advice or treatment |
| 2 | Unmet need | Serious sexual difficulties. Unsafe sex |
| 9 | Not known | |

*If rated 0 or 9 go to Question 18*

### How much help with problems in her sex life does the person receive from partner, friends or relatives?

| Rating | Meaning | Example |
|---|---|---|
| 0 | None | |
| 1 | Low help | Some advice |
| 2 | Moderate help | Several talks, provides information material |
| 3 | High help | Establishes contact with medical or counselling centres and possibly accompanies the person |
| 9 | Not known | |

### How much help with problems in her sex life does the person receive from local services?

### How much help with problems in her sex life does the person need from local services?

| Rating | Meaning | Example |
|---|---|---|
| 0 | None | |
| 1 | Low help | Given information about contraception, safe sex |
| 2 | Moderate help | Regular advice about problems in sex life |
| 3 | High help | Sexual or couple therapy |
| 9 | Not known | |

### User's view of services required

| Action(s) | By whom | Review date |
|---|---|---|
| | | |

# 18 Violence and abuse

### Does the person experience violence or abuse in a current relationship or is she still affected by a previous relationship where she experienced such abuse?

☐ ☐

*Is someone threatening to hurt you or your children?*

*Have you ever been slapped, kicked or punched by someone?*

| Rating | Meaning | Example |
|---|---|---|
| 0 | No need | No issues of violence or abuse |
| 1 | Met need | Has disclosed abuse, receiving counselling |
| 2 | Unmet need (consider impact on child) | Subject to current verbal, physical or sexual abuse or financial exploitation. Past abuse causing current distress |
| 9 | Not known | |

*If rated 0 or 9 go to Question 19*

### How much help does the person receive from partner, friends or relatives for issues of violence and abuse?

☐ ☐

| Rating | Meaning | Example |
|---|---|---|
| 0 | None | |
| 1 | Low help | Able to contact friends or relatives if feeling threatened |
| 2 | Moderate help | Friends or relatives are usually in contact and likely to know if the person is feeling threatened |
| 3 | High help | Friends and relatives are in regular contact and provide a 'safe house' |
| 9 | Not known | |

### How much help does the person receive from local services for issues of violence and abuse?

☐ ☐

### How much help does the person need from local services for issues of violence and abuse?

☐ ☐

| Rating | Meaning | Example |
|---|---|---|
| 0 | None | |
| 1 | Low help | Someone to contact when feeling threatened. Provided with details of domestic violence shelters and programmes |
| 2 | Moderate help | Regular monitoring and support. Help with preparing a personal safety plan |
| 3 | High help | Women's refuge, police protection, victim support |
| 9 | Not known | |

### User's view of services required

| Action(s) | By whom | Review date |
|---|---|---|
| | | |

# 19 Practical demands of childcare

Assessments

User    Staff

## Does the person have any difficulty looking after her child?

*Do you have a child under 16?*

*Do you need any help with parenting?*

| Rating | Meaning | Example |
|---|---|---|
| 0 | No need | No problems looking after child |
| 1 | Met need | Receives and benefiting from advice on child development and parenting |
| 2 | Unmet need (consider impact on child) | Serious difficulties with parenting such as setting boundaries, adequate supervision or effective discipline |
| 8 | Not applicable (not in contact with child) | |
| 9 | Not known | |

*If rated 0 or 9 go to Question 20*

## How much help with looking after the child does the person receive from partner, friends or relatives?

| Rating | Meaning | Example |
|---|---|---|
| 0 | None | |
| 1 | Low help | Occasional child-minding less than once a week, encouragement, advice and support |
| 2 | Moderate help | Regular assistance with parenting or cooperating with access |
| 3 | High help | Child living with partner, friends or relatives. Regular liaison with specialist services |
| 9 | Not known | |

## How much help with looking after her child does the person receive from local services?

## How much help with looking after her child does the person need from local services?

| Rating | Meaning | Example |
|---|---|---|
| 0 | None | |
| 1 | Low help | Provided with parenting books and leaflets |
| 2 | Moderate help | Regular parenting advice or facilitating access |
| 3 | High help | Receiving specialist services, i.e. statutory parenting assessment or intensive parenting classes, child in care |
| 9 | Not known | |

## User's view of services required

| Action(s) | By whom | Review date |
|---|---|---|
| | | |

# 20 Emotional demands of childcare

## Does the person have any diffculties feeling close to her child?

*Do you find it difficult being with your child?*

*Are you affectionate towards your child? How do you express this?*

| Rating | Meaning | Example |
|---|---|---|
| 0 | No need | Displays appropriate affection and warmth |
| 1 | Met need | Counselling helping to develop good mother–child communication |
| 2 | Unmet need (consider impact on child) | Displays unhelpful mother–child communication. Mother is hostile or rejects child |
| 8 | Not applicable (not in contact with child) | |
| 9 | Not known | |

*If rated 0 or 9 go to Question 21*

## How much help does the person receive from partner, friends or relatives with feeling close to her child?

| Rating | Meaning | Example |
|---|---|---|
| 0 | None | |
| 1 | Low help | Some advice from partner, friends or relatives |
| 2 | Moderate help | Regularly monitors and supervises activities with mother–child |
| 3 | High help | Constant support and supervision. Regular liaison with specialist |
| 9 | Not known | |

## How much help does the person receive from local services with feeling close to her child?

## How much help does the person need from local services with feeling close to her child?

| Rating | Meaning | Example |
|---|---|---|
| 0 | None | |
| 1 | Low help | General advice and support |
| 2 | Moderate help | Supervise activities to improve mother–child relationship, i.e. stimulating play, reading, massage, etc. |
| 3 | High help | Referral to specialist services (e.g. CAMHS, Sure Start, etc.), child is removed |
| 9 | Not known | |

## User's view of services required

| Action(s) | By whom | Review date |
|---|---|---|
| | | |

# 21 Basic education

### Does the person lack basic skills in numeracy and literacy?

*Do you have difficulty in reading or writing?*

*Can you count your change in a shop?*

| Rating | Meaning | Example |
|---|---|---|
| 0 | No need | Able to read, write and count |
| 1 | Met need | Assistance provided or attending adult education |
| 2 | Unmet need | Difficulties with basic numeracy and literacy |
| 9 | Not known | |

*If rated 0 or 9 go to Question 22*

### How much help with numeracy and literacy does the person receive from partner, friends or relatives?

| Rating | Meaning | Example |
|---|---|---|
| 0 | None | |
| 1 | Low help | Occasional help to read or write forms |
| 2 | Moderate help | Has put the person in touch with classes |
| 3 | High help | Teaches the person to read, write and count change |
| 9 | Not known | |

### How much help with numeracy and literacy does the person receive from local services?
### How much help help with numeracy and literacy does the person need from local services?

| Rating | Meaning | Example |
|---|---|---|
| 0 | None | |
| 1 | Low help | Help filling in forms |
| 2 | Moderate help | Given advice about classes |
| 3 | High help | Attending adult education |
| 9 | Not known | |

### User's view of services required

| Action(s) | By whom | Review date |
|---|---|---|
| | | |

# 22 Telephone

### Does the person have any difficulty in getting access to or using the telephone?

*Do you have access to a telephone?*

| Rating | Meaning | Example |
|---|---|---|
| 0 | No need | Able to use the telephone and has appropriate access to one |
| 1 | Met need | Has to request use of telephone |
| 2 | Unmet need | No access to telephone or unable to use telephone |
| 9 | Not known | |

*If rated 0 or 9 go to Question 23*

### How much help does the person receive from partner, friends or relatives to make telephone calls?

| Rating | Meaning | Example |
|---|---|---|
| 0 | None | |
| 1 | Low help | Help to make telephone call but less than monthly or only for emergencies |
| 2 | Moderate help | At least weekly help |
| 3 | High help | Daily help if required |
| 9 | Not known | |

### How much help does the person receive from local services to make telephone calls?

### How much help does the person need from local services to make telephone calls?

| Rating | Meaning | Example |
|---|---|---|
| 0 | None | |
| 1 | Low help | Access to telephone upon request |
| 2 | Moderate help | Provided with phonecard |
| 3 | High help | Staff facilitate calls on person's behalf |
| 9 | Not known | |

### User's view of services required

| Action(s) | By whom | Review date |
|---|---|---|
| | | |

# 23 Transport

### Does the person have any problems using public transport?

*Do you have any problems using the bus, tube or train?*

*Do you get a free bus pass?*

| Rating | Meaning | Example |
|---|---|---|
| 0 | No need | Able to use public transport, read timetables or has access to a car |
| 1 | Met need | Bus pass or other help provided with transport |
| 2 | Unmet need | Unable to use public transport or follow timetables |
| 9 | Not known | |

*If rated 0 or 9 go to Question 24*

### How much help with travelling does the person receive from partner, friends or relatives?

| Rating | Meaning | Example |
|---|---|---|
| 0 | None | |
| 1 | Low help | Encouragement to travel |
| 2 | Moderate help | Often accompanies on public transport |
| 3 | High help | Provides transport to all appointments |
| 9 | Not known | |

### How much help with travelling does the person receive from local services?

### How much help with travelling does the person need from local services?

| Rating | Meaning | Example |
|---|---|---|
| 0 | None | |
| 1 | Low help | Provision of bus pass |
| 2 | Moderate help | Taxi card |
| 3 | High help | Transport to appointments by ambulance |
| 9 | Not known | |

### User's view of services required

| Action(s) | By whom | Review date |
|---|---|---|
| | | |

# 24 Budgeting

Assessments

User    Staff

## Does the person have problems budgeting her money?

*How do you find budgeting your money?*

*Do you manage to pay your bills?*

| Rating | Meaning | Example |
|--------|---------|---------|
| 0 | No need | Able to buy essential items and pay bills |
| 1 | Met need | Benefits from help with budgeting |
| 2 | Unmet need | Often has no money for essential items, in serious debt |
| 9 | Not known | |

*If rated 0 or 9 go to Question 25*

## How much help does the person receive from partner, friends or relatives in managing money?

| Rating | Meaning | Example |
|--------|---------|---------|
| 0 | None | |
| 1 | Low help | Occasional help sorting out household bills |
| 2 | Moderate help | Calculating weekly budget |
| 3 | High help | Complete control of finance |
| 9 | Not known | |

## How much help does the person receive from local services in managing money?

## How much help does the person need from local services in managing money?

| Rating | Meaning | Example |
|--------|---------|---------|
| 0 | None | |
| 1 | Low help | Occasional help with budgeting |
| 2 | Moderate help | Supervised in paying rent, given weekly spending money |
| 3 | High help | Daily handouts of cash, in contact with specialist |
| 9 | Not known | |

## User's view of services required

| Action(s) | By whom | Review date |
|-----------|---------|-------------|
| | | |

# 25 Benefits

### Does the person receive all the benefits that she is entitled to?

*Are you sure you are getting all the money you are entitled to?*

| Rating | Meaning | Example |
|---|---|---|
| 0 | No need | Receives full entitlement of benefits |
| 1 | Met need | Receives appropriate help in claiming benefits |
| 2 | Unmet need | Not sure/not receiving full entitlement of benefits |
| 9 | Not known | |

*If rated 0 or 9 go to Question 26*

### How much help does the person receive from partner, friends or relatives in obtaining the full benefit entitlement?

| Rating | Meaning | Example |
|---|---|---|
| 0 | None | |
| 1 | Low help | Occasionally checks whether person is getting money |
| 2 | Moderate help | Has made enquiries about full entitlement |
| 3 | High help | Has helped fill in forms |
| 9 | Not known | |

### How much help does the person receive from local services in obtaining the full benefit entitlement?
### How much help does the person need from local services in obtaining the full benefit entitlement?

| Rating | Meaning | Example |
|---|---|---|
| 0 | None | |
| 1 | Low help | Occasional advice about entitlements |
| 2 | Moderate help | Help with applying for extra entitlements |
| 3 | High help | Comprehensive evaluation of current entitlements |
| 9 | Not known | |

### User's view of services required

| Action(s) | By whom | Review date |
|---|---|---|
| | | |

# 26 Language, culture and religion

Assessments

User    Staff

### Does the person have any specific language, cultural or religious needs?

☐ ☐

*Do you need an interpreter?*

*Do you require any special foods or clothing?*

| Rating | Meaning | Example |
|---|---|---|
| 0 | No need | No needs identified |
| 1 | Met need | Needs identified and arrangements made for interpreter, culturally appropriate diet, etc. |
| 2 | Unmet need | Language barrier. Culturally inappropriate food or no access to place of worship |
| 9 | Not known | |

### How much help does the person receive from partner, friends or relatives with her language, cultural or religious needs?

☐ ☐

| Rating | Meaning | Example |
|---|---|---|
| 0 | None | |
| 1 | Low help | Occasional help |
| 2 | Moderate help | Weekly help with interpreting, meal preparation, praying, etc. |
| 3 | High help | Daily help with interpreting, meal preparation, praying, etc. |
| 9 | Not known | |

### How much help does the person receive from local services with her language, cultural or religious needs?

☐ ☐

### How much help does the person need from local services with her language, cultural or religious needs?

☐ ☐

| Rating | Meaning | Example |
|---|---|---|
| 0 | None | |
| 1 | Low help | Occasional assistance by staff |
| 2 | Moderate help | Assistance at least once per week |
| 3 | High help | Daily assistance with language, cultural or religious needs. Participating in English-speaking classes |
| 9 | Not known | |

### User's view of services required

| Action(s) | By whom | Review date |
|---|---|---|
| | | |

# Appendix 3

# Camberwell Assessment of Need for Mothers (Research version) – CAN–M (R)

# Camberwell Assessment of Need for Mothers (CAN–M)

Assessment date: _____ / _____ / _____
User name/ID: _____
Interviewer: _____

## Child protection issues to consider

When completing the CAN–M questionnaire please give consideration to the impact of the mother's state on the child at all times, especially when unmet needs, or moderate or high help, has been identified in the domains of *Self-care* (4), *Psychotic symptoms* (9), *Psychological distress* (10), *Safety to self* (12), *Safety to child/children and others* (13), *Substance misuse* (14), *Violence and abuse* (18), *Practical demands of childcare* (19), and the *Emotional demands of childcare* (20). If you identify concerns about the impact on the child, then please discuss these concerns with your supervisor or manager. If, after this discussion, you still have concerns and feel that the child and mother would benefit from further services, please speak to the mother's care coordinator. If you consider the child is at suspected or identified risk, however, refer to your local social services.

## Coversheet

(1) Service user

(i) Name: _____ (ii) Date of birth: _____ / _____ / _____

(iii) Contact details:

Address: _____

Home phone: _____ Mobile: _____

(2) Dependants

(i) Is the service user pregnant? Yes / No (please circle correct answer)

(ii) If yes, is the service user attending regular antenatal appointments? Yes / No
(please give details)
_____
_____
_____

(iii) Number of children (under the age of 16 years):

(iv) Age and sex of child/children (youngest to eldest):

Child 1: Age ⬜ Sex ⬜      Child 3: Age ⬜ Sex ⬜      Child 5: Age ⬜ Sex ⬜

Child 2: Age ⬜ Sex ⬜      Child 4: Age ⬜ Sex ⬜      Child 6: Age ⬜ Sex ⬜

(v) Living arrangements of child/children (you may tick more than one option):

Mother ⬜                 Friend ⬜                  Children's home ⬜      Relatives ⬜
Father (if separated) ⬜   Foster family (unrelated) ⬜   Adopted ⬜

(3) Care coordinator

(i) Name: _____ (ii) Title / position: _____

(iii) Contact details: _____

# 1 Accomodation

## Does the person have an appropriate place to live now or following hospital discharge?

*Is your current accommodation appropriate?*

*(If in hospital) Do you have a place to live?*

| Rating | Meaning | Example |
|---|---|---|
| 0 | No need | Accommodation is adequate, secure and childsafe (e.g. child locks, safety gates) |
| 1 | Met need | Person has adequate supported accommodation |
| 2 | Unmet need | Home lacks basic facilities such as water and electricity |
| 9 | Not known | |

*If rated 0 or 9 go to Question 2*

## How much help with accommodation does the person receive from partner, friends or relatives?

| Rating | Meaning | Example |
|---|---|---|
| 0 | None | |
| 1 | Low help | Advice and support |
| 2 | Moderate help | Would provide help with improving accommodation, providing furniture or redecoration |
| 3 | High help | Living with friend/family because own accommodation is unsatisfactory |
| 9 | Not known | |

## How much help with accommodation does the person receive from local services?

## How much help with accommodation will the person need from local services?

| Rating | Meaning | Example |
|---|---|---|
| 0 | None | |
| 1 | Low help | Advice and support |
| 2 | Moderate help | Referral to housing agency for improvements or independent living |
| 3 | High help | Being rehoused, living in group home or hostel |
| 9 | Not known | |

## Does the person receive the right type of help with accommodation?

(0=No; 1=Yes; 9=Not known)

## Overall, is the person satisfied with the amount of help she is receiving with accommodation?

(0=Not satisfied; 1=Satisfied; 9=Not known)

# 2 Food

## Does the person have difficulty in buying and preparing food?

*Are you able to prepare appropriate meals?*

*Are you able to do your own shopping?*

| Rating | Meaning | Example |
|--------|---------|---------|
| 0 | No need | Able to buy and prepare appropriate meals |
| 1 | Met need | Requires assistance to buy or prepare appropriate food, or receives meals |
| 2 | Unmet need | Unable to buy or prepare food or not receiving appropriate help. Diet very limited |
| 9 | Not known | |

*If rated 0 or 9 go to Question 3*

## How much help does the person receive from partner, friends or relatives with buying and preparing food?

| Rating | Meaning | Example |
|--------|---------|---------|
| 0 | None | |
| 1 | Low help | Requires nutritional advice. Weekly prompting or assistance with shopping or food preparation |
| 2 | Moderate help | Daily prompting or assistance with shopping or food preparation |
| 3 | High help | Meals provided daily |
| 9 | Not known | |

## How much help does the person receive from local services with buying and preparing food?

## How much help does the person need from local services with buying and preparing food?

| Rating | Meaning | Example |
|--------|---------|---------|
| 0 | None | |
| 1 | Low help | Requires nutritional advice. Weekly prompting or assistance with shopping or food preparation |
| 2 | Moderate help | Daily prompting or assistance with shopping or food preparation. Attends cooking groups |
| 3 | High help | Meals provided daily |
| 9 | Not known | |

## Does the person receive the right type of help with buying and preparing food?

(0=No; 1=Yes; 9=Not known)

## Overall, is the person satisfied with the amount of help she is receiving with buying and preparing food?

(0=Not satisfied; 1=Satisfied; 9=Not known)

# 3  Looking after the home

## Does the person have difficulty looking after her home?

*Are you able to look after your home or room?*

*Does anyone help you to keep your home/room tidy?*

| Rating | Meaning | Example |
|--------|---------|---------|
| 0 | No need | Keeps home clean and tidy |
| 1 | Met need | Receives and needs regular domestic help |
| 2 | Unmet need | Home is dirty and a potential health hazard |
| 9 | Not known | |

*If rated 0 or 9 go to Question 4*

## How much help does the person receive from partner, friends or relatives with looking after her home?

| Rating | Meaning | Example |
|--------|---------|---------|
| 0 | None | |
| 1 | Low help | Prompts or helps tidy-up occasionally |
| 2 | Moderate help | Prompts or helps clean at least once a week |
| 3 | High help | Supervises the person more than once a week, washes all clothes and cleans the home |
| 9 | Not known | |

## How much help does the person receive from local services with looking after her home?

## How much help does the person need from local services with looking after her home?

| Rating | Meaning | Example |
|--------|---------|---------|
| 0 | None | |
| 1 | Low help | Occasional prompting or assistance by staff |
| 2 | Moderate help | Prompting or assistance at least once a week |
| 3 | High help | Majority of domestic tasks done by staff |
| 9 | Not known | |

## Does the person receive the right type of help with looking after the home?

(0=No; 1=Yes; 9=Not known)

## Overall, is the person satisfied with the amount of help she is receiving with looking after the home?

(0=Not satisfied; 1=Satisfied; 9=Not known)

# 4 Self-care

## Does the person have difficulty with self-care?

*Do you have problems keeping clean and tidy?*

*Do you ever need reminding? Who by?*

| Rating | Meaning | Example |
|---|---|---|
| 0 | No need | Appearance may be unusual, eccentric or untidy, but is basically clean |
| 1 | Met need | Needs and gets help with self-care |
| 2 | Unmet need (consider impact on child) | Poor personel hygiene |
| 9 | Not known | |

*If rated 0 or 9 go to Question 5*

## How much help does the person receive from partner, friends or relatives with self-care?

| Rating | Meaning | Example |
|---|---|---|
| 0 | None | |
| 1 | Low help | Occasionally prompts person to change her clothes, brush her teeth, etc. |
| 2 | Moderate help | Run the bath/shower and insist on its use, daily prompting |
| 3 | High help | Daily assistance with several aspects of self-care |
| 9 | Not known | |

## How much help does the person receive from local services with self-care?

## How much help will the person need from local services with self-care?

| Rating | Meaning | Example |
|---|---|---|
| 0 | None | |
| 1 | Low help | Occasional prompting |
| 2 | Moderate help | Supervise self-care activities |
| 3 | High help | Physically assists with several aspects of self-care or self-care skills programme |
| 9 | Not known | |

## Does the person receive the right type of help with self-care?

(0=No; 1=Yes; 9=Not known)

## Overall, is the person satisfied with the amount of help she is receiving with self-care?

(0=Not satisfied; 1=Satisfied; 9=Not known)

# 5  Daytime activities

## Does the person have difficulty with regular daytime activities?

*How do you spend your day?*

*Do you have enough to do during the day?*

| Rating | Meaning | Example |
|---|---|---|
| 0 | No need | Able to occupy self with work, household, social or childcare activities |
| 1 | Met need | Unable to occupy self, attending occupational therapy or day centre |
| 2 | Unmet need | Not adequately occupied with daytime activities |
| 9 | Not known | |

*If rated 0 or 9 go to Question 6*

## How much help does the person receive from partner, friends or relatives in finding or keeping regular daytime activities?

| Rating | Meaning | Example |
|---|---|---|
| 0 | None | |
| 1 | Low help | Occasional advice about daytime activities |
| 2 | Moderate help | Accompanied to leisure activities |
| 3 | High help | Daily help with arranging daytime activities |
| 9 | Not known | |

## How much help does the person receive from local services in finding or keeping regular daytime activities?
## How much help does the person need from local services in finding or keeping regular daytime activities?

| Rating | Meaning | Example |
|---|---|---|
| 0 | None | |
| 1 | Low help | Advice and information about activities and local facilities |
| 2 | Moderate help | Sheltered employment daily. Attends occupational therapy activities or day centre 2–4 days per week |
| 3 | High help | All daytime activities arranged by staff |
| 9 | Not known | |

## Does the person receive the right type of help with getting daytime activities?

(0=No; 1=Yes; 9=Not known)

## Overall, is the person satisfied with the amount of help she is receiving with daytime activities?

(0=Not satisfied; 1=Satisfied; 9=Not known)

# 6 General physical health

## Does the person have any general physical illness, disability or medication side-effects?

*How do you feel physically?*

*Are you getting treatment for physical problems from your doctor?*

| Rating | Meaning | Example |
|---|---|---|
| 0 | No need | Physically well |
| 1 | Met need | Physical ailment, such as high blood pressure, receiving appropriate treatment |
| 2 | Unmet need | Untreated physical problems, including medication side-effects or ineffective treatment |
| 9 | Not known | |

*If rated 0 or 9 go to Question 7*

## How much help does the person receive from partner, friends or relatives for general physical problems?

| Rating | Meaning | Example |
|---|---|---|
| 0 | None | |
| 1 | Low help | Prompting to see a doctor |
| 2 | Moderate help | Accompanied to medical appointments |
| 3 | High help | Daily help with going to the toilet, eating or mobility |
| 9 | Not known | |

## How much help does the person receive from local services for general physical problems?

## How much help does the person need from local services for general physical problems?

| Rating | Meaning | Example |
|---|---|---|
| 0 | None | |
| 1 | Low help | Given general health advice |
| 2 | Moderate help | Regular review/involvement of specialist medical services (e.g. dietician, GP). Prescribed medication |
| 3 | High help | In-patient or frequent hospital appointments. Alterations to home |
| 9 | Not known | |

## Does the person receive the right type of help for general physical problems?

(0=No; 1=Yes; 9=Not known)

## Overall, is the person satisfied with the amount of help she is receiving for general physical problems?

(0=Not satisfied; 1=Satisfied; 9=Not known)

# 7 Pregnancy care

### Does the person have any physical problems relating to pregnancy or after the birth?

*Do you have any physical problems with your pregnancy?*

*Did you have any birth complications?*

*Are you attending your antenatal appointments?*

| Rating | Meaning | Example |
|---|---|---|
| 0 | No need | Fully recovered from pregnancy and birth |
| 1 | Met need | Receiving appropriate care and monitoring. Attending regular antenatal appointments |
| 2 | Unmet need | Untreated physical problems, including medication side-effects, ineffective treatment or poor antenatal/postnatal care |
| 8 | Not applicable (user is not pregnant or has not recently given birth) | |
| 9 | Not known | |

*If rated 0 or 9 go to Question 8*

### How much help does the person receive from partner, friends or relatives for physical problems relating to pregnancy care?

| Rating | Meaning | Example |
|---|---|---|
| 0 | None | |
| 1 | Low help | Prompting to attend antenatal check-ups |
| 2 | Moderate help | Accompanied to medical appointments |
| 3 | High help | Daily help required owing to physical problems |
| 9 | Not known | |

### How much help does the person receive from local services for physical problems relating to pregnancy care?

### How much help does the person need from local services for problems relating to pregnancy care?

| Rating | Meaning | Example |
|---|---|---|
| 0 | None | |
| 1 | Low help | Given health advice, including dietary advice and breastfeeding information |
| 2 | Moderate help | Involvement of specialist medical services |
| 3 | High help | In-patient or frequent hospital appointments |
| 9 | Not known | |

### Does the person receive the right type of help for physical problems relating to pregnancy?

(0=No; 1=Yes; 9=Not known)

### Overall, is the person satisfied with the amount of help she is receiving for physical problems relating to pregnancy?

(0=Not satisfied; 1=Satisfied; 9=Not known)

# 8 Sleep

## Does the person have any problems with her sleep?

*How well are you sleeping?*

| Rating | Meaning | Example |
|--------|---------|---------|
| 0 | No need | Gets adequate sleep |
| 1 | Met need | Uses sleep aids such as relaxation exercises or music. Shares childcare responsibilities at night |
| 2 | Unmet need | Severely disrupted sleep. Regularly has less than 4 hours per night or unrefreshing sleep |
| 9 | Not known | |

*If rated 0 or 9 go to Question 9*

## How much help does the person receive from partner, friends or relatives for problems with sleep?

| Rating | Meaning | Example |
|--------|---------|---------|
| 0 | None | |
| 1 | Low help | Advice, sympathy and suppport |
| 2 | Moderate help | Prompts the use of sleeping aids. Shares childcare responsibilities at night |
| 3 | High help | Assistance with sleep programme. Family and friends care for child at night |
| 9 | Not known | |

## How much help does the person receive from local services for problems with sleep?

## How much help does the person need from local services for problems with sleep?

| Rating | Meaning | Example |
|--------|---------|---------|
| 0 | None | |
| 1 | Low help | Sleep education |
| 2 | Moderate help | Sleep programme such as the 'controlled crying' technique |
| 3 | High help | Referral to sleep centre. prescribed medication. Hospital staff care for child at night |
| 9 | Not known | |

## Does the person receive the right type of help for problems with sleep?

(0=No; 1=Yes; 9=Not known)

## Overall, is the person satisfied with the amount of help she is receiving for problems with sleep?

(0=Not satisfied; 1=Satisfied; 9=Not known)

# 9 Psychotic symptoms

Assessments

User    Staff

---

**Does the person have any psychotic symptoms such as hallucinations or delusional beliefs?**

*Do you ever hear voices or have problems with your thoughts?*

*Are you on medication or injections? What is it for?*

| Rating | Meaning | Example |
|---|---|---|
| 0 | No need | No positive symptoms, not at risk from symptoms and not on medication |
| 1 | Met need | Symptoms helped by medication or other treatment, e.g. psychological therapy |
| 2 | Unmet need (consider impact on child) | Untreated psychosis/postnatal psychosis or at high risk of relapse |
| 9 | Not known | |

*If rated 0 or 9 go to Question 10*

---

**How much help does the person receive from partner, friends or relatives for these psychotic symptoms?**

| Rating | Meaning | Example |
|---|---|---|
| 0 | None | |
| 1 | Low help | Sympathy and support |
| 2 | Moderate help | Carers involved in helping with coping strategies, relapse prevention and/or medication compliance |
| 3 | High help | Constant supervision of medication, coping strategies and relapse prevention |
| 9 | Not known | |

---

**How much help does the person receive from local services for these psychotic symptoms?**

**How much help does the person need from local services for these psychotic symptoms?**

| Rating | Meaning | Example |
|---|---|---|
| 0 | None | |
| 1 | Low help | Maintenance of medication |
| 2 | Moderate help | Regular review of medication and care plan. Attends support groups or psychotherapy |
| 3 | High help | Medication and 24-hour hospital care or crisis care at home |
| 9 | Not known | |

---

**Does the person receive the right type of help for psychotic symptoms?**

(0=No; 1=Yes; 9=Not known)

**Overall, is the person satisfied with the amount of help she is receiving for psychotic symptoms?**

(0=Not satisfied; 1=Satisfied; 9=Not known)

# 10 Psychological distress

## Does the person suffer from current psychological distress, anxiety or depression?

*Have you recently felt sad or low?*

*Have you felt overly anxious or frightened?*

*Has your mood changed since giving birth?*

| Rating | Meaning | Example |
|---|---|---|
| 0 | No need | Occasional or mild distress |
| 1 | Met need | Receiving appropriate care for anxiety or depression (including post-natal depression) |
| 2 | Unmet need (consider impact on child) | Distress has significant impact on life, i.e. interferes with childcare or work |
| 9 | Not known | |

*If rated 0 or 9 go to Question 11*

## How much help does the person receive from partner, friends or relatives for this distress?

| Rating | Meaning | Example |
|---|---|---|
| 0 | None | |
| 1 | Low help | Some sympathy and support |
| 2 | Moderate help | Opportunity at least weekly to talk about distress to friend or relative |
| 3 | High help | Constant support and supervision |
| 9 | Not known | |

## How much help does the person receive from local services for this distress?

## How much help does the person need from local services for this distress?

| Rating | Meaning | Example |
|---|---|---|
| 0 | None | |
| 1 | Low help | Assessment of mental state or occasional support |
| 2 | Moderate help | Specific psychological or social treatment. Counselled by staff at least once a week |
| 3 | High help | 24-hour hospital care or crisis care |
| 9 | Not known | |

## Does the person receive the right type of help for this distress?

(0=No; 1=Yes; 9=Not known)

## Overall, is the person satisfied with the amount of help she is receiving for this distress?

(0=Not satisfied; 1=Satisfied; 9=Not known)

# 11 Information

## Has the person had clear verbal or written information about her condition, care plan and rights?

*Have you been given clear information about your condition and treatment?*

*Do you understand the role of each professional in your treatment?*

*(Where relevant) Do you know your rights under the Mental Health Act?*

| Rating | Meaning | Example |
|---|---|---|
| 0 | No need | Information retained from previous contact with local services |
| 1 | Met need | Has received and understands sufficient information |
| 2 | Unmet need | Has not received or fails to understand sufficient information. Absence of care plan or pre-birth conference |
| 9 | Not known | |

*If rated 0 or 9 go to Question 12*

## How much help does the person receive from partner, friends or relatives in obtaining such information?

| Rating | Meaning | Example |
|---|---|---|
| 0 | None | |
| 1 | Low help | Some advice given |
| 2 | Moderate help | Given leaflets or put in touch with self-help groups |
| 3 | High help | Regular liaison with doctors or local support groups |
| 9 | Not known | |

## How much help does the person receive from local services in obtaining such information?

## How much help does the person need from local services in obtaining such information?

| Rating | Meaning | Example |
|---|---|---|
| 0 | None | |
| 1 | Low help | Brief verbal or written information |
| 2 | Moderate help | Informal discussions with staff on a range of issues relevant to condition and treatment |
| 3 | High help | Regular structured information sessions with staff to improve knowledge and understanding of condition and treatment |
| 9 | Not known | |

## Does the person receive the right type of help in obtaining information?

(0=No; 1=Yes; 9=Not known)

## Overall, is the person satisfied with the amount of help she is receiving in obtaining information?

(0=Not satisfied; 1=Satisfied; 9=Not known)

# 12 Safety to self

Assessments

User    Staff

---

## Is the person a danger to herself

*Do you ever have thoughts of harming yourself?*

*Have you harmed yourself recently?*

*Do you put yourself in danger in any way?*

| Rating | Meaning | Example |
|---|---|---|
| 0 | No need | Occasional or mild distress |
| 1 | Met need | Needs and receives ongoing support |
| 2 | Unmet need (consider impact on child) | Has expressed suicidal ideas during the last month or has exposed themselves to serious danger |
| 9 | Not known | |

*If rated 0 or 9 go to Question 13*

---

## How much help does the person receive from partner, friends or relatives to reduce the risk of self-harm?

| Rating | Meaning | Example |
|---|---|---|
| 0 | None | |
| 1 | Low help | Able to contact friends or relatives if feeling unsafe |
| 2 | Moderate help | Friends or relatives are usually in contact and are likely to know if person is feeling unsafe |
| 3 | High help | Friends or relatives are in regular contact and would inform staff if disclosed/suspected risk |
| 9 | Not known | |

---

## How much help does the person receive from local services to reduce the risk of self-harm?

## How much help does the person need from local services to reduce the risk of self-harm?

| Rating | Meaning | Example |
|---|---|---|
| 0 | None | |
| 1 | Low help | Someone to contact if feeling unsafe |
| 2 | Moderate help | Staff check at least once a week, receiving supportive counselling |
| 3 | High help | Daily supervision, in-patient care |
| 9 | Not known | |

---

## Does the person receive the right type of help to reduce the risk of self-harm?

(0=No; 1=Yes; 9=Not known)

## Overall, is the person satisfied with the amount of help she is receiving to reduce the risk of self-harm?

(0=Not satisfied; 1=Satisfied; 9=Not known)

# 13 Safety to child/children and others

## Is the person a current or potential risk to her child/children's safety or to other people's safety?

*Do you think you could be a danger to other people's safety?*

*Have you threatened other people or been violent?*

*Do you ever lose your temper and hit your child/children?*

| Rating | Meaning | Example |
|---|---|---|
| 0 | No need | No history of violence or threatening behaviour |
| 1 | Met need | Monitoring risk, receives sufficient appropriate help for this problem |
| 2 | Unmet need (consider impact on child) | Recent harm, violence, threatening behaviour or neglect |
| 9 | Not known | |

*If rated 0 or 9 go to Question 14*

## How much help does the person receive from partner, friends or relatives to reduce the risk that she might harm someone else?

| Rating | Meaning | Example |
|---|---|---|
| 0 | None | |
| 1 | Low help | General advice about threatening behaviour |
| 2 | Moderate help | Support/supervision more than weekly |
| 3 | High help | Daily support/supervision |
| 9 | Not known | |

## How much help does the person receive from local services to reduce the risk that she might harm someone else?

## How much help does the person need from local services to reduce the risk that she might harm someone else?

| Rating | Meaning | Example |
|---|---|---|
| 0 | None | |
| 1 | Low help | Check on behaviour monthly or less, general advice and support |
| 2 | Moderate help | Regular check-ups on behaviour. referral to social services |
| 3 | High help | Constant supervision. Intensive parenting programme. Child removed |
| 9 | Not known | |

## Does the person receive the right type of help to reduce the risk that she might harm someone else?

(0=No; 1=Yes; 9=Not known)

## Overall, is the person satisfied with the amount of help she is receiving to reduce the risk that she might harm someone else?

(0=Not satisfied; 1=Satisfied; 9=Not known)

# 14 Substance misuse

## Does the person have problems with alcohol or drug misuse?

*Does drinking cause you problems?*

*Do you take any drugs that are not prescribed by a doctor?*

*Do you find it difficult to stop?*

| Rating | Meaning | Example |
|--------|---------|---------|
| 0 | No need | No alcohol or drug problem |
| 1 | Met need | At risk from substance misuse and receiving help |
| 2 | Unmet need (consider impact on child) | Harmful and/or uncontrolled use |
| 9 | Not known | |

*If rated 0 or 9 go to Question 15*

## How much help does the person receive from partner, friends or relatives for their substance misuse?

| Rating | Meaning | Example |
|--------|---------|---------|
| 0 | None | |
| 1 | Low help | Encouraged to reduce substance intake |
| 2 | Moderate help | Regular advice, put in contact with helping agencies |
| 3 | High help | Reported concerns to clinical team, working in partnership to reduce intake |
| 9 | Not known | |

## How much help does the person receive from local services for their substance misuse?

## How much help does the person need from local services for their substance misuse?

| Rating | Meaning | Example |
|--------|---------|---------|
| 0 | None | |
| 1 | Low help | Informed about risks, given leaflets |
| 2 | Moderate help | Given details of helping agencies. Counselling |
| 3 | High help | Attends specialist clinic. Supervised withdrawal programme |
| 9 | Not known | |

## Does the person receive the right type of help for substance misuse?

(0=No; 1=Yes; 9=Not known)

## Overall, is the person satisfied with the amount of help she is receiving for substance misuse?

(0=Not satisfied; 1=Satisfied; 9=Not known)

# 15 Company

### Does the person need help with social contact?

*Are you happy with your social life?*

*Do you wish you had more contact with others?*

| Rating | Meaning | Example |
|---|---|---|
| 0 | No need | Able to organise social contact, has enough friends or content with own company |
| 1 | Met need | Attends organised social events, frequently accompanied by support person |
| 2 | Unmet need | Frequently feels lonely and isolated |
| 9 | Not known | |

*If rated 0 or 9 go to Question 16*

### How much help with social contact does the person receive from partner, friends or relatives?

| Rating | Meaning | Example |
|---|---|---|
| 0 | None | |
| 1 | Low help | Social contact less than weekly |
| 2 | Moderate help | Social contact weekly or more often |
| 3 | High help | Social contact at least four times a week |
| 9 | Not known | |

### How much help with social contact does the person receive from local services?

### How much help with social contact does the person need from local services?

| Rating | Meaning | Example |
|---|---|---|
| 0 | None | |
| 1 | Low help | Encourages participation in social activities |
| 2 | Moderate help | Given advice about social clubs or social skills groups |
| 3 | High help | Attends day centre or community group |
| 9 | Not known | |

### Does the person receive the right type of help in organising social contact?

(0=No; 1=Yes; 9=Not known)

### Overall, is the person satisfied with the amount of help she is receiving in organising social contact?

(0=Not satisfied; 1=Satisfied; 9=Not known)

# 16 Intimate relationships

Assessments

User    Staff

### Does the person have any difficulty in starting or maintaining a close relationship?

*Do you have a partner?*

*Do you have problems in your partnership/marriage?*

| Rating | Meaning | Example |
|--------|---------|---------|
| 0 | No need | Satisfactory relationship or content not having a partner |
| 1 | Met need | Receiving helpful advice or therapy |
| 2 | Unmet need | Wants a partner and feels not having one is a problem or unhappy in existing relationship |
| 9 | Not known | |

*If rated 0 or 9 go to Question 17*

### How much help does the person receive from partner, friends or relatives with starting and maintaining close relationships?

| Rating | Meaning | Example |
|--------|---------|---------|
| 0 | None | |
| 1 | Low help | Some support |
| 2 | Moderate help | Regular support and advice. Prompts use of self-help books, etc. |
| 3 | High help | Intensive support in coping with feelings |
| 9 | Not known | |

### How much help does the person receive from local services with starting and maintaining close relationships?

### How much help does the person need from local services with starting and maintaining close relationships?

| Rating | Meaning | Example |
|--------|---------|---------|
| 0 | None | |
| 1 | Low help | Some relationship support |
| 2 | Moderate help | Regular relationship support and advice. Prompts use of self-help books, etc. |
| 3 | High help | Therapy, social skills training |
| 9 | Not known | |

### Does the person receive the right type of help with starting and maintaining close relationships?

(0=No; 1=Yes; 9=Not known)

### Overall, is the person satisfied with the amount of help she is receiving with starting and maintaining close relationships?

(0=Not satisfied; 1=Satisfied; 9=Not known)

# 17 Sexual health

## Does the person have problems with her sex life?

*How is your sex life?*

*Do you require information about safe sex or contraception?*

| Rating | Meaning | Example |
|---|---|---|
| 0 | No need | Content with sex life |
| 1 | Met need | Benefiting from advice or treatment |
| 2 | Unmet need | Serious sexual difficulties. Unsafe sex |
| 9 | Not known | |

*If rated 0 or 9 go to Question 18*

## How much help with problems in her sex life does the person receive from partner, friends or relatives?

| Rating | Meaning | Example |
|---|---|---|
| 0 | None | |
| 1 | Low help | Some advice |
| 2 | Moderate help | Several talks, provides information material |
| 3 | High help | Establishes contact with medical or counselling centres and possibly accompanies the person |
| 9 | Not known | |

## How much help with problems in her sex life does the person receive from local services?

## How much help with problems in her sex life does the person need from local services?

| Rating | Meaning | Example |
|---|---|---|
| 0 | None | |
| 1 | Low help | Given information about contraception, safe sex |
| 2 | Moderate help | Regular advice about problems in sex life |
| 3 | High help | Sexual or couple therapy |
| 9 | Not known | |

## Does the person receive the right type of help for problems in her sex life?

(0=No; 1=Yes; 9=Not known)

## Overall, is the person satisfied with the amount of help she is receiving for problems in her sex life?

(0=Not satisfied; 1=Satisfied; 9=Not known)

# 18 Violence and abuse

**Does the person experience violence or abuse in a current relationship or is she still affected by a previous relationship where she experienced such abuse?**

*Is someone threatening to hurt you or your children?*

*Have you ever been slapped, kicked or punched by someone?*

| Rating | Meaning | Example |
|---|---|---|
| 0 | No need | No issues of violence or abuse |
| 1 | Met need | Has disclosed abuse, receiving counselling |
| 2 | Unmet need (consider impact on child) | Subject to current verbal, physical or sexual abuse or financial exploitation. Past abuse causing current distress |
| 9 | Not known | |

*If rated 0 or 9 go to Question 19*

**How much help does the person receive from partner, friends or relatives for issues of violence and abuse?**

| Rating | Meaning | Example |
|---|---|---|
| 0 | None | |
| 1 | Low help | Able to contact friends or relatives if feeling threatened |
| 2 | Moderate help | Friends or relatives are usually in contact and likely to know if the person is feeling threatened |
| 3 | High help | Friends and relatives are in regular contact and provide a 'safe house' |
| 9 | Not known | |

**How much help does the person receive from local services for issues of violence and abuse?**

**How much help does the person need from local services for issues of violence and abuse?**

| Rating | Meaning | Example |
|---|---|---|
| 0 | None | |
| 1 | Low help | Someone to contact when feeling threatened. Provided with details of domestic violence shelters and programmes |
| 2 | Moderate help | Regular monitoring and support. Help with preparing a personal safety plan |
| 3 | High help | Women's refuge, police protection, victims support |
| 9 | Not known | |

**Does the person receive the right type of help for issues of violence and abuse?**

(0=No; 1=Yes; 9=Not known)

**Overall, is the person satisfied with the amount of help she is receiving for issues of violence and abuse?**

(0=Not satisfied; 1=Satisfied; 9=Not known)

# 19 Practical demands of childcare

## Does the person have any difficulty looking after her child?

*Do you have a child under 16?*

*Do you need any help with parenting?*

| Rating | Meaning | Example |
|--------|---------|---------|
| 0 | No need | No problems looking after child |
| 1 | Met need | Receives and benefiting from advice on child development and parenting |
| 2 | Unmet need (consider impact on child) | Serious difficulties with parenting such as setting boundaries, adequate supervision or effective discipline |
| 8 | Not applicable (not in contact with child) | |
| 9 | Not known | |

*If rated 0 or 9 go to Question 20*

## How much help with looking after the child does the person receive from partner, friends or relatives?

| Rating | Meaning | Example |
|--------|---------|---------|
| 0 | None | |
| 1 | Low help | Occasional child-minding less than once a week, encouragement, advice and support |
| 2 | Moderate help | Regular assistance with parenting or cooperating with access |
| 3 | High help | Child living with partner, friends or relatives. Regular liaison with specialist services |
| 9 | Not known | |

## How much help with looking after her child does the person receive from local services?

## How much help with looking after her child does the person need from local services?

| Rating | Meaning | Example |
|--------|---------|---------|
| 0 | None | |
| 1 | Low help | Provided with parenting books and leaflets |
| 2 | Moderate help | Regular parenting advice or facilitating access |
| 3 | High help | Receiving specialist services, i.e. statutory parenting assessment or intensive parenting classes, child in care |
| 9 | Not known | |

## Does the person receive the right type of help for looking after her child?

(0=No; 1=Yes; 9=Not known)

## Overall, is the person satisfied with the amount of help she is receiving for looking after her child?

(0=Not satisfied; 1=Satisfied; 9=Not known)

# 20 Emotional demands of childcare

Assessments

User     Staff

### Does the person have any diffculties feeling close to her child?

*Do you find it difficult being with your child?*

*Are you affectionate towards your child? How do you express this?*

| Rating | Meaning | Example |
|--------|---------|---------|
| 0 | No need | Displays appropriate affection and warmth |
| 1 | Met need | Counselling helping to develop good mother–child communication |
| 2 | Unmet need (consider impact on child) | Displays unhelpful mother–child communication. Mother is hostile or rejects child |
| 8 | Not applicable (not in contact with child) | |
| 9 | Not known | |

*If rated 0 or 9 go to Question 21*

### How much help does the person receive from partner, friends or relatives with feeling close to her child?

| Rating | Meaning | Example |
|--------|---------|---------|
| 0 | None | |
| 1 | Low help | Some advice from partner, friends or relatives |
| 2 | Moderate help | Regularly monitors and supervises activities with mother–child |
| 3 | High help | Constant support and supervision. Regular liaison with specialist |
| 9 | Not known | |

### How much help does the person receive from local services with feeling close to her child?

### How much help does the person need from local services with feeling close to her child?

| Rating | Meaning | Example |
|--------|---------|---------|
| 0 | None | |
| 1 | Low help | General advice and support |
| 2 | Moderate help | Supervise activities to improve mother–child relationship, i.e. stimulating play, reading, massage, etc. |
| 3 | High help | Referral to specialist services (e.g. CAMHS, Sure Start, etc.), child is removed |
| 9 | Not known | |

### Does the person receive the right type of help with feeling close to her child?

(0=No; 1=Yes; 9=Not known)

### Overall, is the person satisfied with the amount of help she is receiving with feeling close to her child?

(0=Not satisfied; 1=Satisfied; 9=Not known)

# 21 Basic education

## Does the person lack basic skills in numeracy and literacy?

*Do you have difficulty in reading or writing?*

*Can you count your change in a shop?*

| Rating | Meaning | Example |
|---|---|---|
| 0 | No need | Able to read, write and count |
| 1 | Met need | Assistance provided or attending adult education |
| 2 | Unmet need | Difficulties with basic numeracy and literacy |
| 9 | Not known | |

*If rated 0 or 9 go to Question 22*

## How much help with numeracy and literacy does the person receive from partner, friends or relatives?

| Rating | Meaning | Example |
|---|---|---|
| 0 | None | |
| 1 | Low help | Occasional help to read or write forms |
| 2 | Moderate help | Has put the person in touch with classes |
| 3 | High help | Teaches the person to read, write and count change |
| 9 | Not known | |

## How much help with numeracy and literacy does the person receive from local services?

## How much help help with numeracy and literacy does the person need from local services?

| Rating | Meaning | Example |
|---|---|---|
| 0 | None | |
| 1 | Low help | Help filling in forms |
| 2 | Moderate help | Given advice about classes |
| 3 | High help | Attending adult education |
| 9 | Not known | |

## Does the person receive the right type of help with numeracy and literacy?

(0=No; 1=Yes; 9=Not known)

## Overall, is the person satisfied with the amount of help she is receiving with numeracy and literacy?

(0=Not satisfied; 1=Satisfied; 9=Not known)

# 22 Telephone

### Does the person have any difficulty in getting access to or using the telephone?

*Do you have access to a telephone?*

| Rating | Meaning | Example |
|---|---|---|
| 0 | No need | Able to use the telephone and has appropriate access to one |
| 1 | Met need | Has to request use of telephone |
| 2 | Unmet need | No access to telephone or unable to use telephone |
| 9 | Not known | |

*If rated 0 or 9 go to Question 23*

### How much help does the person receive from partner, friends or relatives to make telephone calls?

| Rating | Meaning | Example |
|---|---|---|
| 0 | None | |
| 1 | Low help | Help to make telephone call but less than monthly or only for emergencies |
| 2 | Moderate help | At least weekly help |
| 3 | High help | Daily help if required |
| 9 | Not known | |

### How much help does the person receive from local services to make telephone calls?
### How much help does the person need from local services to make telephone calls?

| Rating | Meaning | Example |
|---|---|---|
| 0 | None | |
| 1 | Low help | Access to telephone upon request |
| 2 | Moderate help | Provided with phonecard |
| 3 | High help | Staff facilitate calls on person's behalf |
| 9 | Not known | |

### Does the person receive the right type of help to make telephone calls?

(0=No; 1=Yes; 9=Not known)

### Overall, is the person satisfied with the amount of help she is receiving to make telephone calls?

(0=Not satisfied; 1=Satisfied; 9=Not known)

# 23 Transport

## Does the person have any problems using public transport?

*Do you have any problems using the bus, tube or train?*

*Do you get a free bus pass?*

| Rating | Meaning | Example |
|--------|---------|---------|
| 0 | No need | Able to use public transport, read timetables or has access to a car |
| 1 | Met need | Bus pass or other help provided with transport |
| 2 | Unmet need | Unable to use public transport or follow timetables |
| 9 | Not known | |

*If rated 0 or 9 go to Question 24*

## How much help with travelling does the person receive from partner, friends or relatives?

| Rating | Meaning | Example |
|--------|---------|---------|
| 0 | None | |
| 1 | Low help | Encouragement to travel |
| 2 | Moderate help | Often accompanies on public transport |
| 3 | High help | Provides transport to all appointments |
| 9 | Not known | |

## How much help with travelling does the person receive from local services?

## How much help with travelling does the person need from local services?

| Rating | Meaning | Example |
|--------|---------|---------|
| 0 | None | |
| 1 | Low help | Provision of bus pass |
| 2 | Moderate help | Taxi card |
| 3 | High help | Transport to appointments by ambulance |
| 9 | Not known | |

## Does the person receive the right type of help with travelling?

(0=No; 1=Yes; 9=Not known)

## Overall, is the person satisfied with the amount of help she is receiving with travelling?

(0=Not satisfied; 1=Satisfied; 9=Not known)

# 24 Budgeting

## Does the person have problems budgeting her money?

*How do you find budgeting your money?*

*Do you manage to pay your bills?*

| Rating | Meaning | Example |
|---|---|---|
| 0 | No need | Able to buy essential items and pay bills |
| 1 | Met need | Benefits from help with budgeting |
| 2 | Unmet need | Often has no money for essential items, in serious debt |
| 9 | Not known | |

*If rated 0 or 9 go to Question 25*

## How much help does the person receive from partner, friends or relatives in managing money?

| Rating | Meaning | Example |
|---|---|---|
| 0 | None | |
| 1 | Low help | Occasional help sorting out household bills |
| 2 | Moderate help | Calculating weekly budget |
| 3 | High help | Complete control of finance |
| 9 | Not known | |

## How much help does the person receive from local services in managing money?

## How much help does the person need from local services in managing money?

| Rating | Meaning | Example |
|---|---|---|
| 0 | None | |
| 1 | Low help | Occasional help with budgeting |
| 2 | Moderate help | Supervised in paying rent, given weekly spending money |
| 3 | High help | Daily handouts of cash, in contact with specialist |
| 9 | Not known | |

## Does the person receive the right type of help in managing her money?

(0=No; 1=Yes; 9=Not known)

## Overall, is the person satisfied with the amount of help she is receiving in managing her money?

(0=Not satisfied; 1=Satisfied; 9=Not known)

# 25 Benefits

### Does the person receive all the benefits that she is entitled to?

*Are you sure you are getting all the money you are entitled to?*

| Rating | Meaning | Example |
|--------|---------|---------|
| 0 | No need | Receives full entitlement of benefits |
| 1 | Met need | Receives appropriate help in claiming benefits |
| 2 | Unmet need | Not sure/not receiving full entitlement of benefits |
| 9 | Not known | |

*If rated 0 or 9 go to Question 26*

### How much help does the person receive from partner, friends or relatives in obtaining the full benefit entitlement?

| Rating | Meaning | Example |
|--------|---------|---------|
| 0 | None | |
| 1 | Low help | Occasionally checks whether person is getting money |
| 2 | Moderate help | Has made enquiries about full entitlement |
| 3 | High help | Has helped fill in forms |
| 9 | Not known | |

### How much help does the person receive from local services in obtaining the full benefit entitlement?

### How much help does the person need from local services in obtaining the full benefit entitlement?

| Rating | Meaning | Example |
|--------|---------|---------|
| 0 | None | |
| 1 | Low help | Occasional advice about entitlements |
| 2 | Moderate help | Help with applying for extra entitlements |
| 3 | High help | Comprehensive evaluation of current entitlements |
| 9 | Not known | |

### Does the person receive the right type of help in obtaining the full benefit entitlement?

(0=No; 1=Yes; 9=Not known)

### Overall, is the person satisfied with the amount of help she is receiving in obtaining the full benefit entitlement?

(0=Not satisfied; 1=Satisfied; 9=Not known)

# 26 Language, culture and religion

## Does the person have any specific language, cultural or religious needs?

*Do you need an interpreter?*

*Do you require any special foods or clothing?*

| Rating | Meaning | Example |
|---|---|---|
| 0 | No need | No needs identified |
| 1 | Met need | Needs identified and arrangements made for interpreter, culturally appropriate diet, etc. |
| 2 | Unmet need | Language barrier. Culturally inappropriate food or no access to place of worship |
| 9 | Not known | |

## How much help does the person receive from partner, friends or relatives with her language, cultural or religious needs?

| Rating | Meaning | Example |
|---|---|---|
| 0 | None | |
| 1 | Low help | Occasional help |
| 2 | Moderate help | Weekly help with interpreting, meal preparation, praying, etc. |
| 3 | High help | Daily help with interpreting, meal preparation, praying, etc. |
| 9 | Not known | |

## How much help does the person receive from local services with her language, cultural or religious needs?

## How much help does the person need from local services with her language, cultural or religious needs?

| Rating | Meaning | Example |
|---|---|---|
| 0 | None | |
| 1 | Low help | Occasional assistance by staff |
| 2 | Moderate help | Assistance at least once per week |
| 3 | High help | Daily assistance with language, cultural or religious needs. Participating in English-speaking classes |
| 9 | Not known | |

## Does the person receive the right type of help with her language, cultural or religious needs?

(0=No; 1=Yes; 9=Not known)

## Overall, is the person satisfied with the amount of help she is receiving with her language, cultural or religious needs?

(0=Not satisfied; 1=Satisfied; 9=Not known)

# Appendix 4

# Camberwell Assessment of Need for Mothers (Short Appraisal Schedule version) – CAN–M (S)

# CAN–M (S) – Short version

| User name: _____ | | 0=No problem | 1=Met need | 2=Unmet need |
| Name of assessor: _____ | Date of assessment: ___ / ___ / ___ | 8=Not applicable** | 9=Not known | |

| Circle who is interviewed (U=User, S=Staff) | U | S |
|---|---|---|
| **1. Accommodation** <br> Does the person have an appropriate place to live now or following hospital discharge? | | |
| **2. Food** <br> Does the person have difficulty in buying and preparing food? | | |
| **3. Looking after the home** <br> Does the person have difficulty looking after her home? | | |
| **4. Self-care** <br> Does the person have difficulty with self-care? | | |
| **5. Daytime activities** <br> Does the person have difficulty with regular daytime activities? | | |
| **6. General physical health** <br> Does the person have any general physical illness, disability or medication side-effects? | | |
| **7. Pregnancy care**\*\* <br> Does the person have any physical problem relating to pregnancy or after the birth? | | |
| **8. Sleep** <br> Does the person have any problems with her sleep? | | |
| **9. Psychotic symptoms** <br> Does the person have any psychotic symptoms such as hallucinations or delusional beliefs? | | |
| **10. Psychological distress** <br> Does the person suffer from current psychological distress, anxiety or depression? | | |
| **11. Information** <br> Has the person had clear verbal or written information about her condition, care plan and rights? | | |
| **12. Safety to self** <br> Is the person a danger to herself? | | |
| **13. Safety to child/children and others** <br> Is the person a current or potential risk to her child/children's safety or to other people's safety? | | |
| **14. Substance misuse** <br> Does the person have problems with alcohol or drug misuse? | | |
| **15. Company** <br> Does the person need help with social contact? | | |
| **16. Intimate relationships** <br> Does the person have any difficulty in starting or maintaining a close relationship? | | |
| **17. Sexual health** <br> Does the person have problems with her sex life? | | |
| **18. Violence and abuse** <br> Does the person experience violence or abuse in a current relationship or is she still affected by a previous relationship where she experienced such abuse? | | |
| **19. Practical demands of childcare**\*\* <br> Does the person have any difficulty looking after her child? | | |
| **20. Emotional demands of childcare**\*\* <br> Does the person have any difficulties feeling close to her child? | | |
| **21. Basic education** <br> Does the person lack basic skills in numeracy and literacy? | | |
| **22. Telephone** <br> Does the person have any difficulty in getting access to or using the telephone? | | |
| **23. Transport** <br> Does the person have any problems using public transport? | | |
| **24. Budgeting** <br> Does the person have problems budgeting her money? | | |
| **25. Benefits** <br> Does the person receive all the benefits that she is entitled to? | | |
| **26. Language, culture and religion** <br> Does the person have specific language, cultural or religious needs? | | |

| | | |
|---|---|---|
| **A – Met needs** (count the number of 1s in the column) | | |
| **B – Unmet needs** (count the number of 2s in the column) | | |
| **C – Total number of needs** (add together A and B) | | |

© *The Royal College of Psychiatrists, 2008. This page may be photocopied freely.*

# Appendix 5

## CAN–M (C) Assessment summary score sheets

These score sheets summarise the data collected during a CAN–M (C) interview, giving a condensed record of the full interview. Complete and separate user and staff summary score sheets are available.

The CAN–M (S) is a self-contained document, and so does not need a separate summary sheet.

# CAN–M (C)
# Complete assessment summary sheet

User name: _____     Date of assessment: _____ / _____ / _____

Interviewer's name: _____     Date of last review: _____ / _____ / _____

| User/Staff rating | Section 1 Need identified | | Section 2 Informal help given | | Section 3 Formal help given | | Section 3 Formal help needed | | User's views recorded | Action plan? |
|---|---|---|---|---|---|---|---|---|---|---|
| **Rating** | 0, 1, 2, 8, 9 | | 0, 1, 2, 3, 9 | | 0, 1, 2, 3, 9 | | 0, 1, 2, 3, 9 | | Yes | Review date |
| **User/Staff rating** | U | S | U | S | U | S | U | S | U | S |
| 1.  Accommodation | | | | | | | | | | |
| 2.  Food | | | | | | | | | | |
| 3.  Looking after the home | | | | | | | | | | |
| 4.  Self-care | | | | | | | | | | |
| 5.  Daytime activities | | | | | | | | | | |
| 6.  General physical health | | | | | | | | | | |
| 7.  Pregnancy care | | | | | | | | | | |
| 8.  Sleep | | | | | | | | | | |
| 9.  Psychotic symptoms | | | | | | | | | | |
| 10. Psychological distress | | | | | | | | | | |
| 11. Information | | | | | | | | | | |
| 12. Safety to self | | | | | | | | | | |
| 13. Safety to child/children and others | | | | | | | | | | |
| 14. Substance misuse | | | | | | | | | | |
| 15. Company | | | | | | | | | | |
| 16. Intimate relationships | | | | | | | | | | |
| 17. Sexual health | | | | | | | | | | |
| 18. Violence and abuse | | | | | | | | | | |
| 19. Practical demands of childcare | | | | | | | | | | |
| 20. Emotional demands of childcare | | | | | | | | | | |
| 21. Basic education | | | | | | | | | | |
| 22. Telephone | | | | | | | | | | |
| 23. Transport | | | | | | | | | | |
| 24. Budgeting | | | | | | | | | | |
| 25. Benefits | | | | | | | | | | |
| 26. Language, culture and religion | | | | | | | | | | |
| **Number of met needs** (Number of 1s) | | | | | | | | | | |
| **Number of unmet needs** (Number of 2s) | | | | | | | | | | |
| **Total number of needs** (Number of 1s and 2s) | | | | | | | | | | |
| **Total level of help given and needed** (Add scores, rate 9 as 0) | | | | | | | | | | |

# CAN–M (C)
# User assessment summary sheet

User name: _____    Date of assessment: ____ / ____ / ____

Interviewer's name: _____    Date of last review: ____ / ____ / ____

| Rating | Need identified<br>0, 1, 2, 8, 9 | Informal help given<br>0, 1, 2, 3, 9 | Formal help given<br>0, 1, 2, 3, 9 | Formal help needed<br>0, 1, 2, 3, 9 | User's views recorded<br>Yes | Action plan?<br>Review date |
|---|---|---|---|---|---|---|
| 1. Accommodation | | | | | | |
| 2. Food | | | | | | |
| 3. Looking after the home | | | | | | |
| 4. Self-care | | | | | | |
| 5. Daytime activities | | | | | | |
| 6. General physical health | | | | | | |
| 7. Pregnancy care | | | | | | |
| 8. Sleep | | | | | | |
| 9. Psychotic symptoms | | | | | | |
| 10. Psychological distress | | | | | | |
| 11. Information | | | | | | |
| 12. Safety to self | | | | | | |
| 13. Safety to child/children and others | | | | | | |
| 14. Substance misuse | | | | | | |
| 15. Company | | | | | | |
| 16. Intimate relationships | | | | | | |
| 17. Sexual health | | | | | | |
| 18. Violence and abuse | | | | | | |
| 19. Practical demands of childcare | | | | | | |
| 20. Emotional demands of childcare | | | | | | |
| 21. Basic education | | | | | | |
| 22. Telephone | | | | | | |
| 23. Transport | | | | | | |
| 24. Budgeting | | | | | | |
| 25. Benefits | | | | | | |
| 26. Language, culture and religion | | | | | | |
| **Number of met needs** (Number of 1s) | | | | | | |
| **Number of unmet needs** (Number of 2s) | | | | | | |
| **Total number of needs** (Number of 1s and 2s) | | | | | | |
| **Total level of help given and needed** (Add scores, rate 9 as 0) | | | | | | |

*© The Royal College of Psychiatrists, 2008. This page may be photocopied freely.*

# CAN–M (C)
# Staff assessment summary sheet

User name: _____   Date of assessment: _____ / _____ / _____
Interviewer's name: _____   Date of last review: _____ / _____ / _____

| | Need identified | Informal help given | Formal help given | Formal help needed | Action plan? |
|---|---|---|---|---|---|
| Rating | 0, 1, 2, 8, 9 | 0, 1, 2, 3, 9 | 0, 1, 2, 3, 9 | 0, 1, 2, 3, 9 | Review date |
| 1.  Accommodation | | | | | |
| 2.  Food | | | | | |
| 3.  Looking after the home | | | | | |
| 4.  Self-care | | | | | |
| 5.  Daytime activities | | | | | |
| 6.  General physical health | | | | | |
| 7.  Pregnancy care | | | | | |
| 8.  Sleep | | | | | |
| 9.  Psychotic symptoms | | | | | |
| 10. Psychological distress | | | | | |
| 11. Information | | | | | |
| 12. Safety to self | | | | | |
| 13. Safety to child/children and others | | | | | |
| 14. Substance misuse | | | | | |
| 15. Company | | | | | |
| 16. Intimate relationships | | | | | |
| 17. Sexual health | | | | | |
| 18. Violence and abuse | | | | | |
| 19. Practical demands of childcare | | | | | |
| 20. Emotional demands of childcare | | | | | |
| 21. Basic education | | | | | |
| 22. Telephone | | | | | |
| 23. Transport | | | | | |
| 24. Budgeting | | | | | |
| 25. Benefits | | | | | |
| 26. Language, culture and religion | | | | | |
| **Number of met needs** (Number of 1s) | | | | | |
| **Number of unmet needs** (Number of 2s) | | | | | |
| **Total number of needs** (Number of 1s and 2s) | | | | | |
| **Total level of help given and needed** (Add scores, rate 9 as 0) | | | | | |

# Appendix 6

## CAN–M (R) Assessment summary score sheet

This score sheet summarises the data collected during a CAN–M (R) interview, giving a condensed record of the full interview.

The CAN–M (S) is a self-contained document, and so does not need a separate summary sheet.

# CAN–M (R)
# Complete assessment summary sheet

User name: _____   Date of assessment: ____ / ____ / ____

Interviewer's name: _____   Date of last review: ____ / ____ / ____

| | Section 1 Need identified | | Section 2 Informal help given | | Section 3 Formal help given | | Section 3 Formal help needed | | Section 4 Type of help | | Section 4 Amount of help |
|---|---|---|---|---|---|---|---|---|---|---|---|
| **Rating** | 0, 1, 2, 8 or 9 | | 0, 1, 2, 3 or 9 | | 0, 1, 2, 3 or 9 | | 0, 1, 2, 3 or 9 | | 0, 1 or 9 | | 0, 1 or 9 |
| **User/Staff rating** | U | S | U | S | U | S | U | S | U | S | S |
| 1. Accommodation | | | | | | | | | | | |
| 2. Food | | | | | | | | | | | |
| 3. Looking after the home | | | | | | | | | | | |
| 4. Self-care | | | | | | | | | | | |
| 5. Daytime activities | | | | | | | | | | | |
| 6. General physical health | | | | | | | | | | | |
| 7. Pregnancy care | | | | | | | | | | | |
| 8. Sleep | | | | | | | | | | | |
| 9. Psychotic symptoms | | | | | | | | | | | |
| 10. Psychological distress | | | | | | | | | | | |
| 11. Information | | | | | | | | | | | |
| 12. Safety to self | | | | | | | | | | | |
| 13. Safety to child/children and others | | | | | | | | | | | |
| 14. Substance misuse | | | | | | | | | | | |
| 15. Company | | | | | | | | | | | |
| 16. Intimate relationships | | | | | | | | | | | |
| 17. Sexual health | | | | | | | | | | | |
| 18. Violence and abuse | | | | | | | | | | | |
| 19. Practical demands of childcare | | | | | | | | | | | |
| 20. Emotional demands of childcare | | | | | | | | | | | |
| 21. Basic education | | | | | | | | | | | |
| 22. Telephone | | | | | | | | | | | |
| 23. Transport | | | | | | | | | | | |
| 24. Budgeting | | | | | | | | | | | |
| 25. Benefits | | | | | | | | | | | |
| 26. Language, culture and religion | | | | | | | | | | | |
| **Number of met needs** (Number of 1s) | | | | | | | | | | | |
| **Number of unmet needs** (Number of 2s) | | | | | | | | | | | |
| **Total number of needs** (Number of 1s and 2s) | | | | | | | | | | | |
| **Total level of help given and needed** (Add scores, rate 9 as 0) | | | | | | | | | | | |

# Appendix 7

# Training overheads

# Training session

## 1 The Camberwell Assessment of Need for Mothers (CAN–M)

### Aims of the session:
What are needs?
Why assess needs?
Benefits of using the CAN–M
CAN–M administration and scoring
Important issues to consider

# 2 Needs assessment in pregnant women and mothers with severe mental illness

- Definition of need and importance of needs assessment

  'The requirements of individuals to enable them to achieve, maintain and restore an acceptable level of social independence or quality of life'

  (National Health Service and Community Care Act 1990)

- Services should be provided on the basis of need

- Everyone has needs arising from a variety of causes

- Need as a subjective concept

- Pregnant women and mothers with severe mental illness have specific needs that may not be met by current services

# 3 Benefits of using the CAN–M

- Brief and user-friendly

- Comprehensive (26 domains)

- Incorporates both service user and staff views

- Records met and unmet needs

- Measures the help provided by informal supports and services separately

- Valid and reliable

- No formal training

- Suitable for research and clinical use

# 4 CAN–M: need domains

1. Accommodation
2. Food
3. Looking after the home
4. Self-care
5. Daytime activities
6. General physical health
7. Pregnancy care
8. Sleep
9. Psychotic symptoms
10. Psychological distress
11. Information
12. Safety to self
13. Safety to child/children and others
14. Substance misuse
15. Company
16. Intimate relationships
17. Sexual health
18. Violence and abuse
19. Practical demands of childcare
20. Emotional demands of childcare
21. Basic education
22. Transport
23. Telephone
24. Budget
25. Benefits
26. Language, culture and religion

# 5 Introducing the CAN–M coversheet

- Information is collected about the service user, her children and the care coordinator

- The impact of the mother's mental state on the child must be considered *at all times*

- There is a need to break confidentiality if a child is thought to be at risk of harm

- Care coordinators and social workers are suitable professionals to contact if child protection issues are identified

# 6  Introducing the four CAN–M sections

## Met and unmet needs

### *Section 1*

- Acts as a filter to determine the need for further assessment and provides an overall needs rating for the domain

    i.  A need is met if the person has no problem or a mild to moderate problem in the domain, owing to the help given (rating 1)

    ii.  A need is unmet if the person has a current serious problem in the domain, irrespective of help given (rating 2)

    iii.  There is no need if the person has no problem in the domain and no help is given (rating 0)

    iv.  The rating is not known if the person does not know or does not wish to answer (rating 9)

    v.  The question is not applicable to the service user (rating 8)

# 7 Introducing the four CAN–M sections

## Help and satisfaction

### Section 2

- Assesses how much informal help from partner, friends and relatives has been received during the past month

Rating key is identical for Sections 2 and 3:

0 = no help
1 = low help
2 = moderate help
3 = high help
9 = not known

### Section 3

- Assesses current and required levels of support from services. It rates perceived levels of help received and the interviewee's perception of what help she actually needs

# 7 Introducing the four CAN–M sections

## Help and satisfaction (continued)

### *Section 4*

*CAN–M (C)*
- Records any other information

- Records action plan

*CAN–M (R)*
- Assesses the user's overall satisfaction with the help she is currently receiving

  Rating key:

  0 = not satisfied
  1 = satisfied
  9 = not known

# 8 Other issues to consider when assessing the needs of pregnant women and mothers with severe mental illness

- Motherhood is often an integral part of identity

- Fear of custody loss

- History of abuse

- Support of partner and extended family

- Involvement of specialist services, e.g. social services, perinatal services

- Stigma

# 9 Scoring

- Summary score sheets

    i.   Met needs (count the number of 1s)

    ii.  Unmet needs (count the number of 2s)

    iii. Total needs (add number of met and unmet needs)

    iv.  Total level of help given, needed and level of satisfaction (add scores, rate 9 and 8 as 0)

# 10 Case vignettes: rating needs using CAN–M (S)

- Read the vignettes

- Identify the needs according to the user and staff

- Discuss whether the domains included are:

  i.   No need
  ii.  Met need
  iii. Unmet need
  iv.  Not applicable
  v.   Not known

- Where do staff and user views differ and how would you address the discrepancies?

# 11  Case vignettes: rating levels of help using CAN–M (R)

- Read the vignettes for the domains of *Pregnancy care, Safety to child/children and others,* and *Emotional demands of childcare*

- Identify the levels of support from formal and informal care, and whether the help provided is the right type and amount

- Where do staff and user views differ and how would you address the discrepancies?

# Appendix 8

# Training vignettes

(a) Three CAN–M (S) practice vignettes and summary score sheets are provided for rating needs.

(b) Three CAN–M (R) practice vignettes are provided for rating (1) the levels of informal and formal support given, and (2) whether the user is receiving the right type of help and whether she is satisfied with the amount of help given. The completed summary scores are provided for the three domains of *Pregnancy care*, *Safety to child/children and others*, and *Emotional demands of childcare*. These vignettes are also suitable for CAN–M (C).

# Three practice vignettes with the CAN–M (S)

## First case vignette

*Nosira – Service user's account*

My name is Nosira and I am 22 years old. My husband and I came to London almost 2 years ago from Bangladesh. When we first arrived here we stayed with his family until we found a place of our own. But our new home is not good – it has mould on the walls, problems with the water supply and no telephone.

I was first admitted to hospital soon after our arrival in this country. I was very worried that people were spying on me and other times I thought that the radio was sending me special messages. I was told I had a mental illness and given medication and I now feel better. I do my shopping and look after the home. However, although I am able to read, write and count money in my own language, I am not able to do this in English. I also cannot read train timetables and so I have difficulty travelling on public transport. My goal is to start attending English-speaking classes in the next few weeks and Lema has told me about local classes. I hope that I will meet other women in my situation there. At the moment I am rather bored, lonely and isolated. I have been married to my husband now for almost 5 years but sometimes when he gets really angry with me he will shout at me and hit me. Sometimes I feel so sad I cry myself to sleep. I am not very happy in my marriage. My husband keeps all the money we get from the state but he gives me enough to buy food for us. I am now 6 months pregnant with my first child and I go to my antenatal clinic regularly (my husband's family are always reminding me to attend my antenatal appointments). At first I was a bit worried about having a child while on medication, but my nurse, Lema, has reassured me that my baby will be fine and I need the medication. I don't have any side-effects with my medication.

*Lema – Keyworker's account*

Nosira is a 22 year-old Bangladeshi woman who migrated to London 2 years ago. She and her husband are currently living in a one-bedroom apartment which lacks basic amenities such as running water and a telephone line. I first came into contact with Nosira several weeks after she was discharged from her first hospital admission. Nosira has a psychotic illness and although she has never been thought of as a risk to others, when she is unwell she has been known to put herself at risk by not eating. Nosira is 6 months pregnant with her first child and she is doing very well. She has not missed a single antenatal appointment and her general physical health and sleep are very good. At one stage Nosira showed some initial reluctance to take her mediation while pregnant, but after discussing the benefits of her continuing to take it, she has agreed to continue on medication for at least another year. Nosira is able to take good care of the family home, prepare her own meals, and to take care of her own personal hygiene and appearance. She does not use any illegal substances and has up-to-date information on her care plan. I do not think she is experiencing any psychotic symptoms at present.

Nosira has very limited English reading and writing skills. She has shown a genuine interest to improve her English skills and would like to be referred to a language course. She has problems using public transport owing to her limited English reading skills and I therefore visit her at home. She has told me that she often feels bored during the day and that she would like to socialise with people other than her in-laws. Although Nosira does not talk about her husband very often it is clear to me that there is significant tension between the two of them. I am also becoming quite concerned about the possibility that there may be some domestic violence in the relationship.

# Completed summary scores for CAN–M (S): first case vignette

| | | |
|---|---|---|
| **User name**: Nosira | 0=No problem    1=Met need    2=Unmet need | |
| **Name of assessor**: Lema Davis, primary nurse    **Date of assessment**: 08 / 10 / 04 | 8=Not applicable**    9=Not known | |

| Circle who is interviewed (U=User, S=Staff) | U | S |
|---|---|---|
| **1. Accommodation** <br> Does the person have an appropriate place to live now or following hospital discharge? | 2 | 2 |
| **2. Food** <br> Does the person have difficulty in buying and preparing food? | 0 | 0 |
| **3. Looking after the home** <br> Does the person have difficulty looking after her home? | 0 | 0 |
| **4. Self-care** <br> Does the person have difficulty with self-care? | 0 | 0 |
| **5. Daytime activities** <br> Does the person have difficulty with regular daytime activities? | 2 | 2 |
| **6. General physical health** <br> Does the person have any general physical illness, disability or medication side-effects? | 0 | 0 |
| **7. Pregnancy care**\*\* <br> Does the person have any physical problem relating to pregnancy or after the birth? | 1 | 1 |
| **8. Sleep** <br> Does the person have any problems with her sleep? | 0 | 0 |
| **9. Psychotic symptoms** <br> Does the person have any psychotic symptoms such as hallucinations or delusional beliefs? | 1 | 1 |
| **10. Psychological distress** <br> Does the person suffer from current psychological distress, anxiety or depression? | 2 | 9 |
| **11. Information** <br> Has the person had clear verbal or written information about her condition, care plan and rights? | 1 | 1 |
| **12. Safety to self** <br> Is the person a danger to herself? | 0 | 1 |
| **13. Safety to child/children and others** <br> Is the person a current or potential risk to her child/children's safety or to other people's safety? | 9 | 0 |
| **14. Substance misuse** <br> Does the person have problems with alcohol or drug misuse? | 0 | 0 |
| **15. Company** <br> Does the person need help with social contact? | 2 | 2 |
| **16. Intimate relationships** <br> Does the person have any difficulty in starting or maintaining a close relationship? | 2 | 2 |
| **17. Sexual health** <br> Does the person have problems with her sex life? | 0 | 9 |
| **18. Violence and abuse** <br> Does the person experience violence or abuse in a current relationship or is she still affected by a previous relationship where she experienced such abuse? | 2 | 9 |
| **19. Practical demands of childcare**\*\* <br> Does the person have any difficulty looking after her child? | 8 | 8 |
| **20. Emotional demands of childcare**\*\* <br> Does the person have any difficulties feeling close to her child? | 8 | 8 |
| **21. Basic education** <br> Does the person lack basic skills in numeracy and literacy? | 0 | 0 |
| **22. Telephone** <br> Does the person have any difficulty in getting access to or using the telephone? | 2 | 2 |
| **23. Transport** <br> Does the person have any problems using public transport? | 2 | 2 |
| **24. Budgeting** <br> Does the person have problems budgeting her money? | 0 | 0 |
| **25. Benefits** <br> Does the person receive all the benefits that she is entitled to? | 0 | 0 |
| **26. Language, culture and religion** <br> Does the person have specific language, cultural or religious needs? | 2 | 2 |

| | | |
|---|---|---|
| **A – Met needs** (count the number of 1s in the column) | 3 | 4 |
| **B – Unmet needs** (count the number of 2s in the column) | 9 | 7 |
| **C – Total number of needs** (add together A and B) | 12 | 11 |

# Second case vignette

## Samantha – Service user's account

I would say I am an unhappy person. I often have thoughts about harming myself and hear some scary voices in my head. The staff at the hospital are always telling me to take better care of myself and to tidy my room, but I don't feel I can; I feel too awful. I feel physically sick every morning because of the medication I am taking and because of my sleepless nights. The activities on offer at the hospital do not interest me, nor does the food but at least I get three meals every day here. I do not have the energy to do anything other than watch TV. I do get pretty lonely but have always struggled to make new friends. I am the mother of two children. My children were removed from my care 6 years ago after social services decided that I was not fit to care for them. I do not have any contact with them. Sometimes I feel this is unbearable, and I tend to drink most days to make me feel a bit better, though this can lead to physical fights. I haven't had a partner in about 2 years and have not had sex in over 12 months but would rather not anyway. I was abused as a child, so I find sexual relationships difficult. Nobody ever wants to talk about the abuse I suffered as a child and it seems impossible to get help with this. I do not really understand why I am in hospital. The information given to me is confusing and I don't really understand how long they intend to keep me in here. I am desperate to be discharged so I can return home. I wish they had a second phone in the ward as there is often a long queue to use it. I would also like to visit the hospital chaplain but I don't know where he is. And I need to see a welfare officer as I do not really know if I am receiving all the benefits I am entitled to and I am always struggling with debt. I can look after myself though – I did well at school and get out and about without any problems.

## James – Keyworker's account

Samantha is a 30-year-old woman who was admitted to our ward 3 weeks ago with delusional beliefs and hallucinations. Staff are monitoring these psychotic symptoms. Samantha tends to display fairly poor personal hygiene and requires prompting by friends and family, as well as staff to supervise self-care activities. Her room is often found to be in a dirty and untidy state despite receiving daily help from staff. Samantha does very little during the day and describes experiencing a lot of psychological symptoms which do not appear to improve with staff support. She reports nausea which may be due to her medication, and has been encouraged to stop sleeping during the day in an attempt to improve her night-time sleep. Samantha frequently reports that she does not understand why she is in hospital, despite receiving regular information about her condition and treatment plan. She has reported daily use of alcohol when outside of hospital and says that this is the main cause for all her debts, which have spiralled out of control. Samantha has two children aged 7 and 10 years of age. They were placed in the care of Samantha's biological mother several years ago.

Samantha reports that she often feels lonely and isolated, despite people's attempts to include her in social activities. She does not have a partner, which makes her feel sad. She also has a history of being abused as a child but says that she does not want to talk about this, though I think she would benefit from some help dealing with her past. Samantha has adequate reading and writing skills, appropriate access to a telephone, and is able to use public transport without any difficulties. She is also receiving all the benefits she is entitled to. She does not have any language, culture or religious needs. She will return to supported housing upon hospital discharge.

# Completed summary scores for CAN–M (S): second case vignette

| | | |
|---|---|---|
| **User name:** Samantha | 0=No problem | 1=Met need 2=Unmet need |
| **Name of assessor:** James Jones, social worker **Date of assessment:** 27 / 04 / 04 | 8=Not applicable** | 9=Not known |

| Circle who is interviewed (U=User, S=Staff) | U | S |
|---|---|---|
| 1. **Accommodation** <br> Does the person have an appropriate place to live now or following hospital discharge? | 1 | 1 |
| 2. **Food** <br> Does the person have difficulty in buying and preparing food? | 1 | 1 |
| 3. **Looking after the home** <br> Does the person have difficulty looking after her home? | 0 | 2 |
| 4. **Self-care** <br> Does the person have difficulty with self-care? | 0 | 1 |
| 5. **Daytime activities** <br> Does the person have difficulty with regular daytime activities? | 2 | 2 |
| 6. **General physical health** <br> Does the person have any general physical illness, disability or medication side-effects? | 2 | 2 |
| 7. **Pregnancy care**** <br> Does the person have any physical problem relating to pregnancy or after the birth? | 8 | 8 |
| 8. **Sleep** <br> Does the person have any problems with her sleep? | 2 | 1 |
| 9. **Psychotic symptoms** <br> Does the person have any psychotic symptoms such as hallucinations or delusional beliefs? | 2 | 2 |
| 10. **Psychological distress** <br> Does the person suffer from current psychological distress, anxiety or depression? | 2 | 2 |
| 11. **Information** <br> Has the person had clear verbal or written information about her condition, care plan and rights? | 2 | 2 |
| 12. **Safety to self** <br> Is the person a danger to herself? | 2 | 2 |
| 13. **Safety to child/children and others** <br> Is the person a current or potential risk to her child/children's safety or to other people's safety? | 2 | 9 |
| 14. **Substance misuse** <br> Does the person have problems with alcohol or drug misuse? | 2 | 2 |
| 15. **Company** <br> Does the person need help with social contact? | 2 | 2 |
| 16. **Intimate relationships** <br> Does the person have any difficulty in starting or maintaining a close relationship? | 2 | 2 |
| 17. **Sexual health** <br> Does the person have problems with her sex life? | 2 | 9 |
| 18. **Violence and abuse** <br> Does the person experience violence or abuse in a current relationship or is she still affected by a previous relationship where she experienced such abuse? | 2 | 2 |
| 19. **Practical demands of childcare**** <br> Does the person have any difficulty looking after her child? | 8 | 8 |
| 20. **Emotional demands of childcare**** <br> Does the person have any difficulties feeling close to her child? | 8 | 8 |
| 21. **Basic education** <br> Does the person lack basic skills in numeracy and literacy? | 0 | 0 |
| 22. **Telephone** <br> Does the person have any difficulty in getting access to or using the telephone? | 2 | 0 |
| 23. **Transport** <br> Does the person have any problems using public transport? | 0 | 0 |
| 24. **Budgeting** <br> Does the person have problems budgeting her money? | 2 | 2 |
| 25. **Benefits** <br> Does the person receive all the benefits that she is entitled to? | 2 | 0 |
| 26. **Language, culture and religion** <br> Does the person have specific language, cultural or religious needs? | 2 | 0 |

| | | |
|---|---|---|
| **A – Met needs** (count the number of 1s in the column) | 2 | 4 |
| **B – Unmet needs** (count the number of 2s in the column) | 17 | 12 |
| **C – Total number of needs** (add together A and B) | 19 | 16 |

© *The Royal College of Psychiatrists, 2008. This page may be photocopied freely.*

# Third case vignette

## Julianne – Service user's account

I am a mother of a 2-month-old daughter, Haley. Before my pregnancy I worked as a shop assistant but I was made redundant 1 year ago. Three weeks ago I was taken to hospital after hearing some very frightening voices which told me to kill myself. I have been told that these voices are part of an illness, which was triggered by my pregnancy and the birth of my child. I had some initial problems with feeling close to my baby daughter and knowing how to care for her but I have been participating in regular sessions with the nursery nurses and now feel much more confident and capable of taking care of her emotionally and practically. Since coming here I have had a lot of support from the staff, who have helped to look after myself – to have daily showers, to clean my room and to eat regularly – and have given me a lot of information about my illness. The occupational therapist has encouraged me to take part in dance therapy, art classes and baby massage. Although I do not have any physical health problems, I do seem to have a lot of trouble falling asleep at night and I never feel refreshed when I wake up in the morning. I have been with my partner Terry now for almost 5 years, and although we argue, I do find him very supportive and a good father. Our sex life is 'non-existent' at the moment inevitably, but I am sure our sex life will return when I feel better. Terry and I have had a lot of difficulties in managing our budget, though we are currently receiving financial counselling from a voluntary organisation to help us pay back our debts. I have been told I may also be eligible for the Disability Living Allowance. I drive our car, though I am not sure if I will be able to on my new medication, so I suppose I will have to use public transport for a while, and I have a mobile phone. I would describe myself as being only a social drinker, and although I can get really anxious at times, I now know that I am well on the road to recovery. I will be returning to our rented apartment once discharged from hospital and I have many good friends to turn to for support.

## Kim – Keyworker's account

Julianne was admitted to hospital voluntarily 3 weeks ago following the onset of a post-natal psychosis and thoughts of self-harm. Medication was prescribed upon admission and the side-effects of her medication appear to be minimal. She presents as being a fairly sociable person on the ward and has made some remarkable improvements in her self-care, ability to keep her room tidy and participation in daytime activities, although she still requires prompting and encouragement in these areas. However, she has days when she feels quite low and worries about her ability to cope once she is discharged from hospital. Her low mood seems to be quite responsive to general staff support and advice though. Although Julianne had some initial attachment problems with her daughter, the staff have helped her spend time with her baby and she now displays appropriate ways of caring, bathing, stimulating and playing with her daughter. Physically, Julianne is doing quite well and she is certainly eating much better than before admission. She has no history of being a risk to self, of abusing drugs, or of being a risk to others. Julianne's partner Terry appears to be very supportive of her needs, and has advised us that Julianne usually has a busy life and supportive friends. They have had a good sexual relationship, which they expect to return to in the near future. Julianne appears to be making good progress in paying back her outstanding debts, and has requested some assistance in knowing whether she is eligible for the Disability Living Allowance. I will look into this for her. Julianne has a good education and has no problem using the telephone and public transport. She has appropriate accommodation and does not have any particular cultural or religious needs.

# Completed summary scores for CAN–M (S): third case vignette

**User name**: Julianne

**Name of assessor**: Kim Cooper, psychologist     **Date of assessment**: 12 / 06 / 05

0=No problem     1=Met need     2=Unmet need

8=Not applicable**     9=Not known

| Circle who is interviewed (U=User, S=Staff) | U | S |
|---|---|---|
| **1. Accommodation** <br> Does the person have an appropriate place to live now or following hospital discharge? | 0 | 0 |
| **2. Food** <br> Does the person have difficulty in buying and preparing food? | 1 | 1 |
| **3. Looking after the home** <br> Does the person have difficulty looking after her home? | 1 | 1 |
| **4. Self-care** <br> Does the person have difficulty with self-care? | 1 | 1 |
| **5. Daytime activities** <br> Does the person have difficulty with regular daytime activities? | 1 | 1 |
| **6. General physical health** <br> Does the person have any general physical illness, disability or medication side-effects? | 0 | 0 |
| **7. Pregnancy care**** <br> Does the person have any physical problem relating to pregnancy or after the birth? | 0 | 0 |
| **8. Sleep** <br> Does the person have any problems with her sleep? | 2 | 9 |
| **9. Psychotic symptoms** <br> Does the person have any psychotic symptoms such as hallucinations or delusional beliefs? | 1 | 1 |
| **10. Psychological distress** <br> Does the person suffer from current psychological distress, anxiety or depression? | 1 | 1 |
| **11. Information** <br> Has the person had clear verbal or written information about her condition, care plan and rights? | 1 | 1 |
| **12. Safety to self** <br> Is the person a danger to herself? | 1 | 1 |
| **13. Safety to child/children and others** <br> Is the person a current or potential risk to her child/children's safety or to other people's safety? | 0 | 0 |
| **14. Substance misuse** <br> Does the person have problems with alcohol or drug misuse? | 0 | 0 |
| **15. Company** <br> Does the person need help with social contact? | 0 | 0 |
| **16. Intimate relationships** <br> Does the person have any difficulty in starting or maintaining a close relationship? | 0 | 0 |
| **17. Sexual health** <br> Does the person have problems with her sex life? | 0 | 0 |
| **18. Violence and abuse** <br> Does the person experience violence or abuse in a current relationship or is she still affected by a previous relationship where she experienced such abuse? | 0 | 0 |
| **19. Practical demands of childcare**** <br> Does the person have any difficulty looking after her child? | 1 | 1 |
| **20. Emotional demands of childcare**** <br> Does the person have any difficulties feeling close to her child? | 1 | 1 |
| **21. Basic education** <br> Does the person lack basic skills in numeracy and literacy? | 0 | 0 |
| **22. Telephone** <br> Does the person have any difficulty in getting access to or using the telephone? | 0 | 0 |
| **23. Transport** <br> Does the person have any problems using public transport? | 0 | 0 |
| **24. Budgeting** <br> Does the person have problems budgeting her money? | 1 | 1 |
| **25. Benefits** <br> Does the person receive all the benefits that she is entitled to? | 2 | 2 |
| **26. Language, culture and religion** <br> Does the person have specific language, cultural or religious needs? | 0 | 0 |

| | U | S |
|---|---|---|
| **A – Met needs** (count the number of 1s in the column) | 11 | 11 |
| **B – Unmet needs** (count the number of 2s in the column) | 2 | 1 |
| **C – Total number of needs** (add together A and B) | 13 | 12 |

© *The Royal College of Psychiatrists, 2008. This page may be photocopied freely.*

# Three practice vignettes with the CAN–M (R)/CAN–M (C)

## Pregnancy care

*Caroline – Service user's account*

I regularly attend my antenatal appointments and medication reviews. My partner, Dave, is very supportive and regularly takes time off work to accompany me to these appointments. This pregnancy has been fairly uneventful compared to my last two, and sometimes I wonder if I really need to attend all of the medical tests that are scheduled for me by the doctors. But I do feel that the medical staff are taking exceptionally good care of me during this pregnancy.

*Dr Smith – GP's account*

My client, Caroline, is very good at attending all of her medical appointments and seems to receive a significant amount of support from her partner, such as accompanying her to medical appointments. Owing to physical complications in previous pregnancies, Caroline has received appropriate additional monitoring from a number of special medical services.

## CAN–M (R)
## User assessment summary sheet

User name: Caroline  Date of assessment: 24 / 05 / 05
Interviewer's name: Dr Smith, GP  Date of last review: ___ / ___ / ___

| | Need identified | Informal help given | Formal help given | Formal help needed | Type of help | Amount of help |
|---|---|---|---|---|---|---|
| **Rating** | 0, 1, 2, 8 or 9 | 0, 1, 2, 3 or 9 | 0, 1, 2, 3 or 9 | 0, 1, 2, 3 or 9 | 0, 1 or 9 | 0, 1 or 9 |
| 7. Pregnancy care | 1 | 2 | 2 | 1 | 1 | 1 |

## CAN–M (R)
## Staff assessment summary sheet

User name: Caroline  Date of assessment: 24 / 05 / 05
Interviewer's name: Dr Smith, GP  Date of last review: ___ / ___ / ___

| | Need identified | Informal help given | Formal help given | Formal help needed | Type of help |
|---|---|---|---|---|---|
| **Rating** | 0, 1, 2, 8 or 9 | 0, 1, 2, 3 or 9 | 0, 1, 2, 3 or 9 | 0, 1, 2, 3 or 9 | 0, 1 or 9 |
| 7. Pregnancy care | 1 | 2 | 2 | 2 | 1 |

## Safety to child/children and others

*Sophie – Service user's account*

My name is Sophie and I am 34 years old. I am the mother of three children who are currently living with their grandmother as I have been told I am unfit to care for them. I do not think I am any risk to my children and think that there has been a misunderstanding between the local authorities and myself. I hope the children will be returned to me soon.

*Chris – Keyworker's account*

Sophie has recently had her children removed from her care due to an excessive use of corporal punishment (e.g. hitting, verbally abusing). Her mother is currently looking after them. I am currently in the process of referring her for a parenting programme.

## CAN–M (R)
## User assessment summary sheet

| User name: Sophie | Date of assessment: 03 / 06 / 05 |
|---|---|
| Interviewer's name: Chris Peters, nurse | Date of last review: _____ / _____ / _____ |

|  | Need identified | Informal help given | Formal help given | Formal help needed | Type of help | Amount of help |
|---|---|---|---|---|---|---|
| **Rating** | **0, 1, 2, 8 or 9** | **0, 1, 2, 3 or 9** | **0, 1, 2, 3 or 9** | **0, 1, 2, 3 or 9** | **0, 1 or 9** | **0, 1 or 9** |
| 13. Safety to child/children and others | 0 | 3 | 3 | 0 | 0 | 0 |

## CAN–M (R)
## Staff assessment summary sheet

| User name: Sophie | Date of assessment: 03 / 06 / 05 |
|---|---|
| Interviewer's name: Chris Peters, nurse | Date of last review: _____ / _____ / _____ |

|  | Need identified | Informal help given | Formal help given | Formal help needed | Type of help |
|---|---|---|---|---|---|
| **Rating** | **0, 1, 2, 8 or 9** | **0, 1, 2, 3 or 9** | **0, 1, 2, 3 or 9** | **0, 1, 2, 3 or 9** | **0, 1 or 9** |
| 13. Safety to child/children and others | 2 | 3 | 3 | 3 | 0 |

# Emotional demands of childcare

*Fiona – Service user's account*

I have a 6-week-old baby which is the result of an unplanned pregnancy. I do not feel prepared to look after a baby and at times I feel uncomfortable being with my child. I have considered adoption on a number of occasions and will be seeing someone from social services later this week to discuss my options. My mother regularly comes to visit me and helps me with childcare activities. I am only getting a small amount of help from social services; maybe my daughter and I would be better off if she was put in care as I am not coping.

*Helen – Keyworker's account*

Although Fiona has expressed some difficulties in feeling emotionally close to her child, she is receiving help with this and the relationship has improved substantially over the past month. Her mother regularly comes to visit and help out, and Fiona also receives general advice and support from myself and her health visitor for improving her communication with the child. I believe she is now receiving the right level of support from local services to meet her needs.

# CAN–M (R)
## User assessment summary sheet

**User name**: Fiona  **Date of assessment**: 30 / 09 / 05
**Interviewer's name**: Helen Hall, nurse  **Date of last review**: _____ / _____ / _____

| | Need identified | Informal help given | Formal help given | Formal help needed | Type of help | Amount of help |
|---|---|---|---|---|---|---|
| **Rating** | **0, 1, 2, 8 or 9** | **0, 1, 2, 3 or 9** | **0, 1, 2, 3 or 9** | **0, 1, 2, 3 or 9** | **0, 1 or 9** | **0, 1 or 9** |
| 20. Emotional demands of childcare | 2 | 2 | 1 | 3 | 0 | 0 |

# CAN–M (R)
## Staff assessment summary sheet

**User name**: Fiona  **Date of assessment**: 30 / 09 / 05
**Interviewer's name**: Helen Hall, nurse  **Date of last review**: _____ / _____ / _____

| | Need identified | Informal help given | Formal help given | Formal help needed | Type of help |
|---|---|---|---|---|---|
| **Rating** | **0, 1, 2, 8 or 9** | **0, 1, 2, 3 or 9** | **0, 1, 2, 3 or 9** | **0, 1, 2, 3 or 9** | **0, 1 or 9** |
| 20. Emotional demands of childcare | 1 | 2 | 2 | 1 | 1 |